MAY 2022

PICTURE BOOK OF FLOWERS

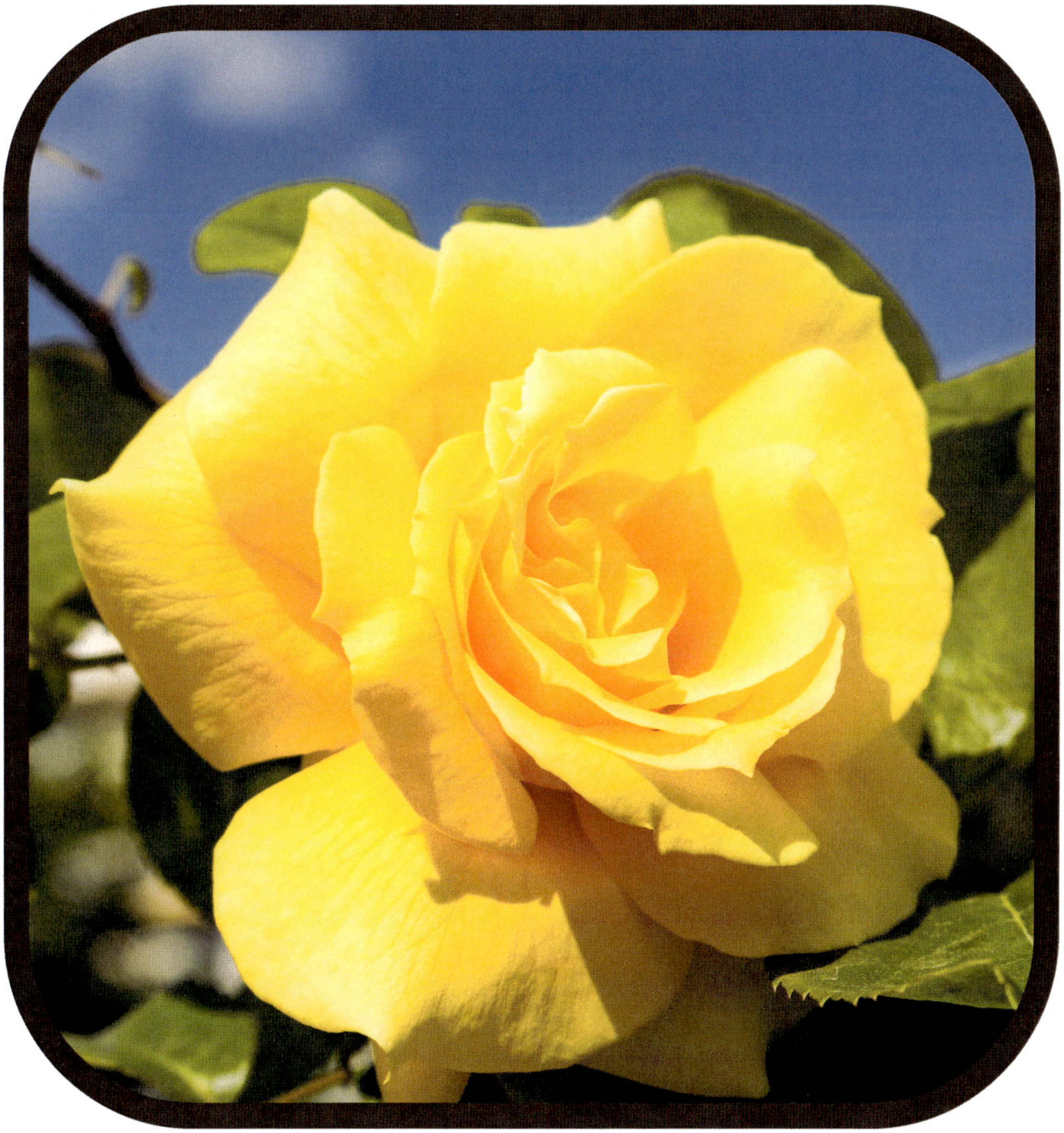

Copyright Books That Matter

BLEEDING HEART

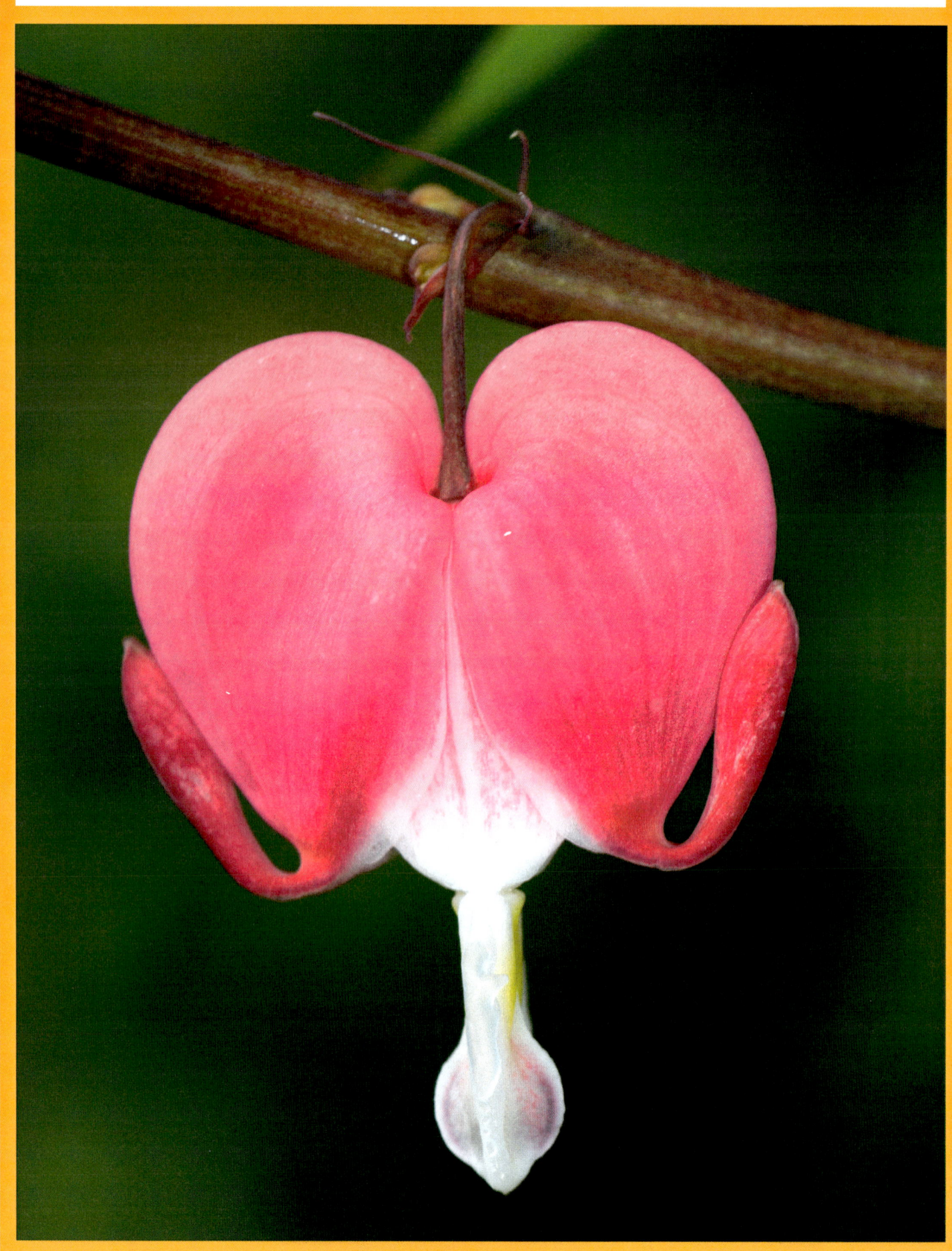

CHRYSANTHEMUM

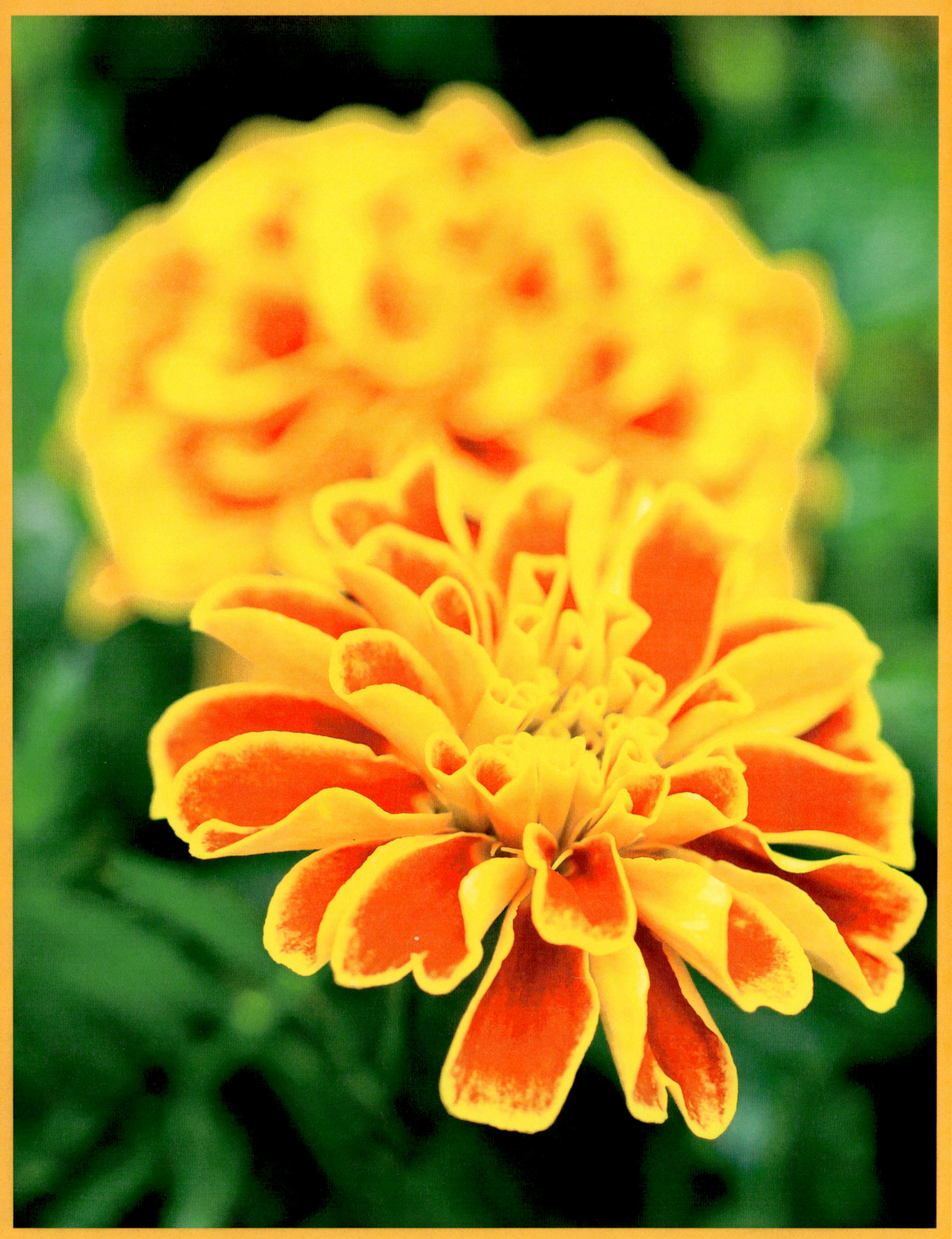

DAHLIA

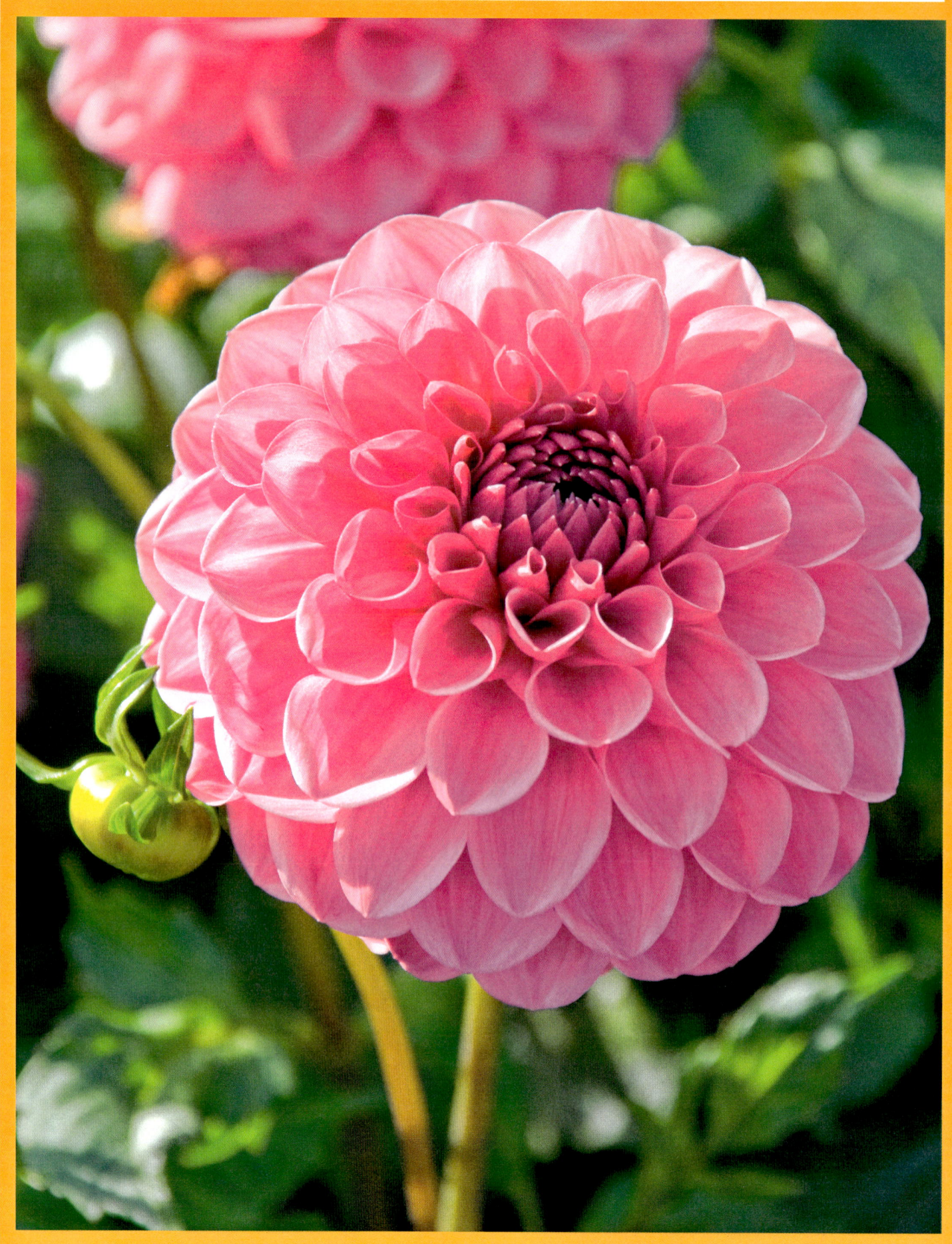

ALLIUM

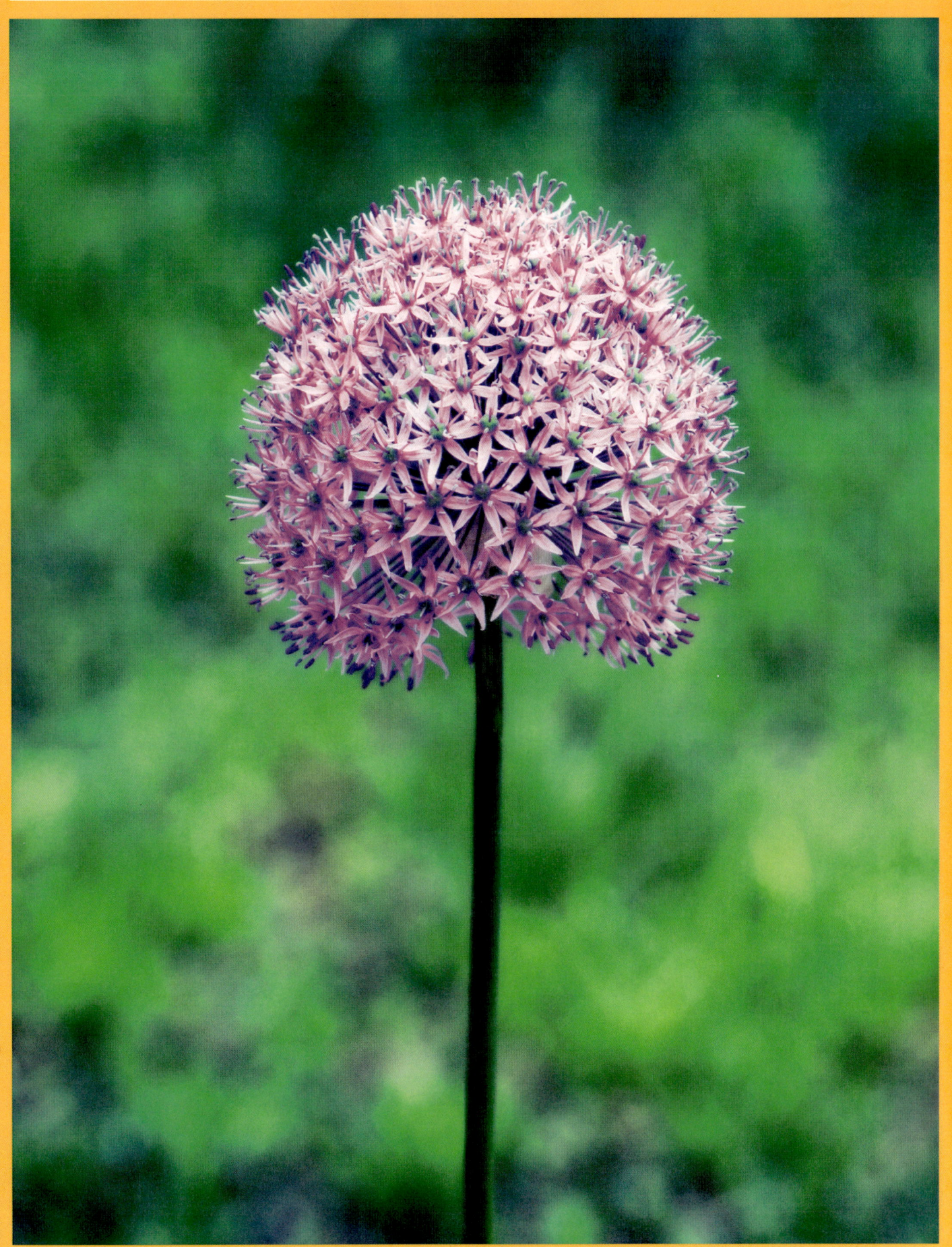

CHRIST FLOWER

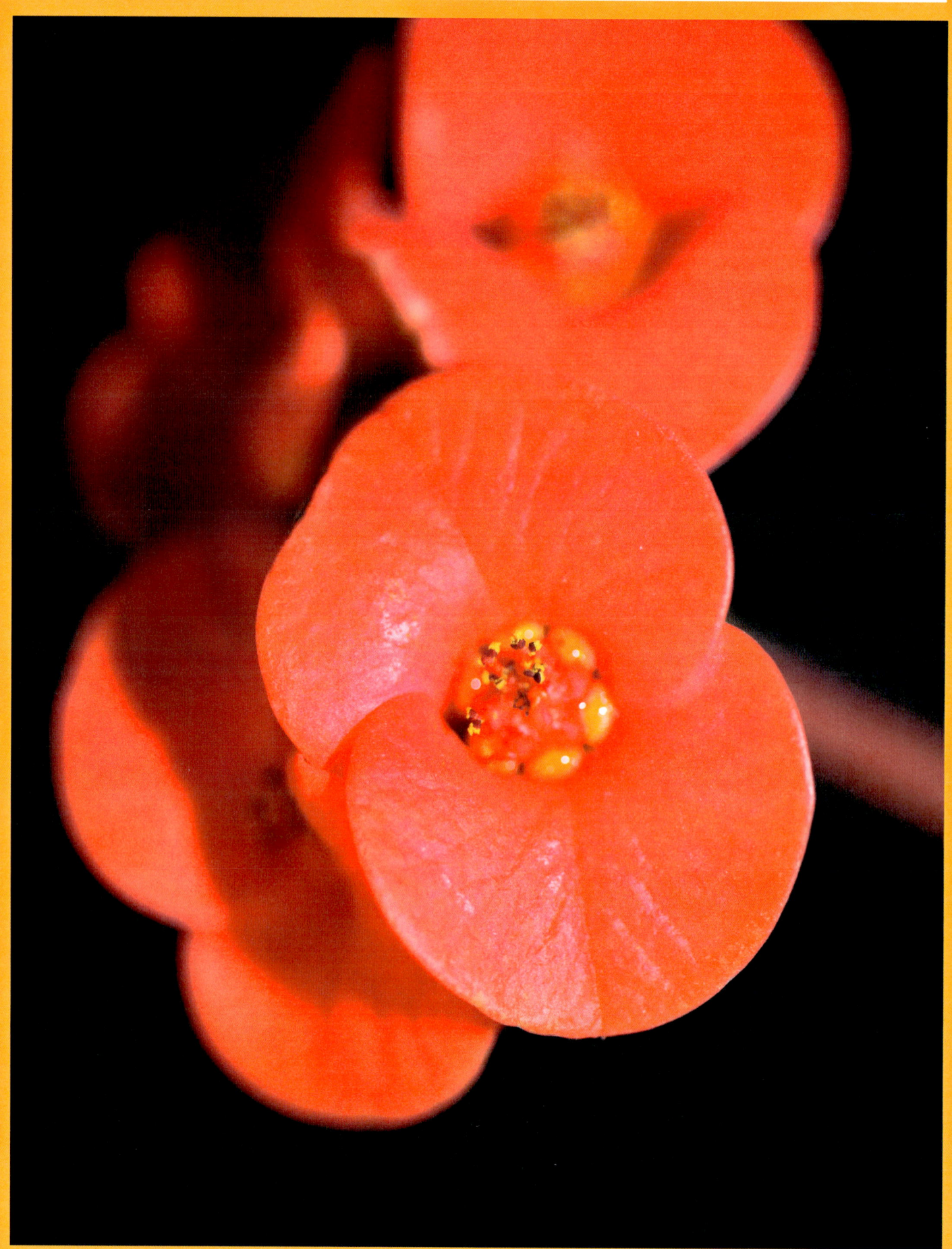

DAYLILY

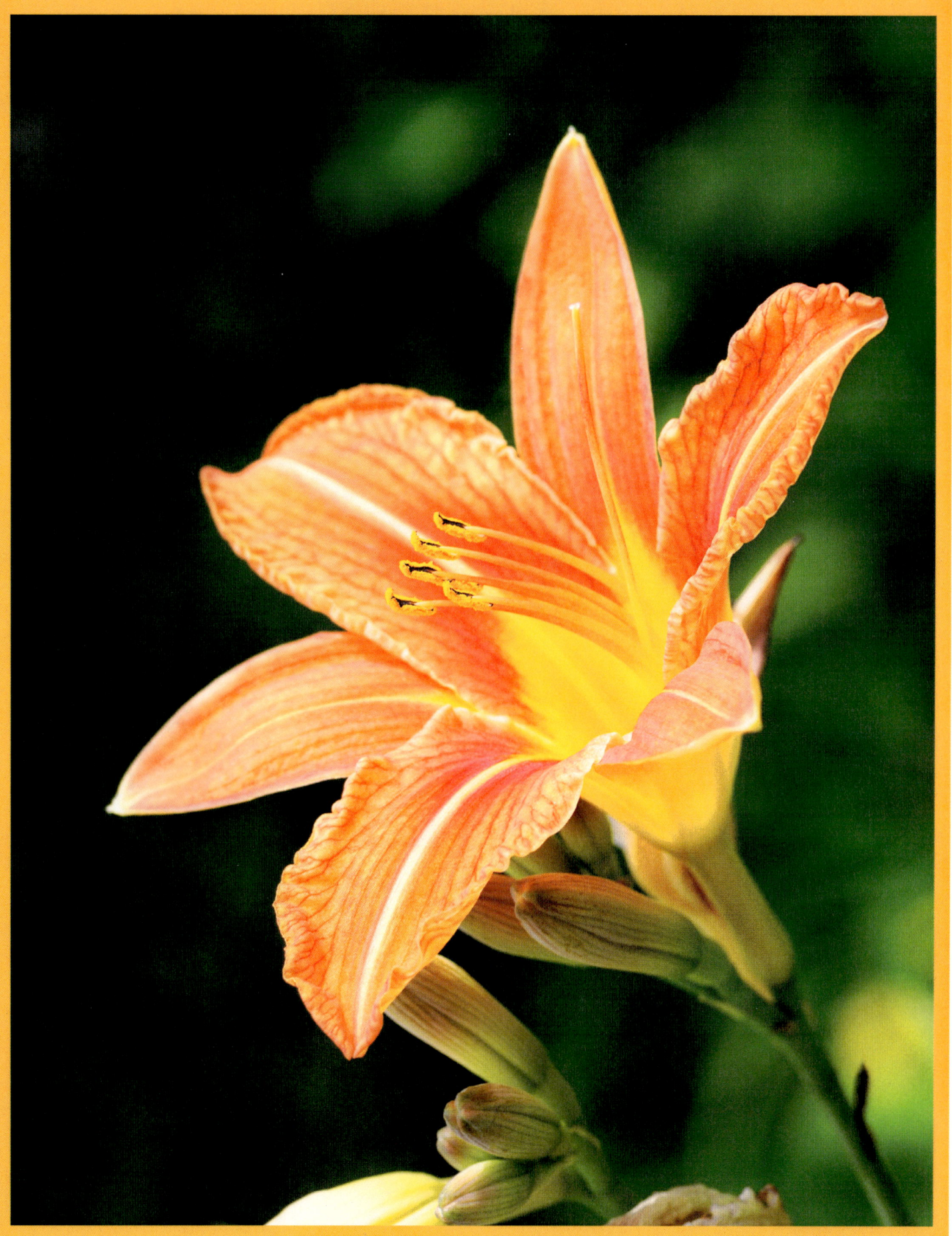

APPLE BLOSSOM

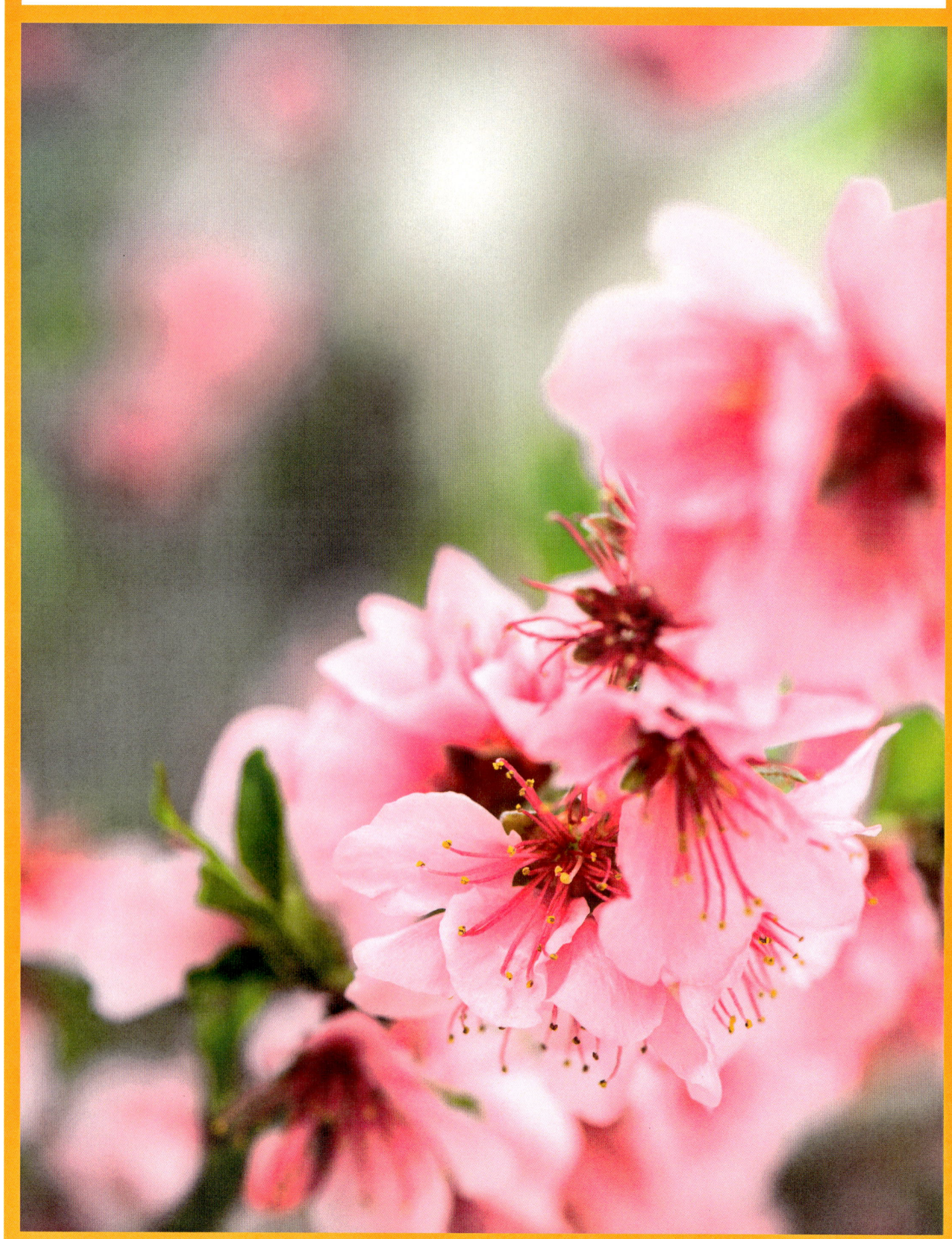

DAFFODIL

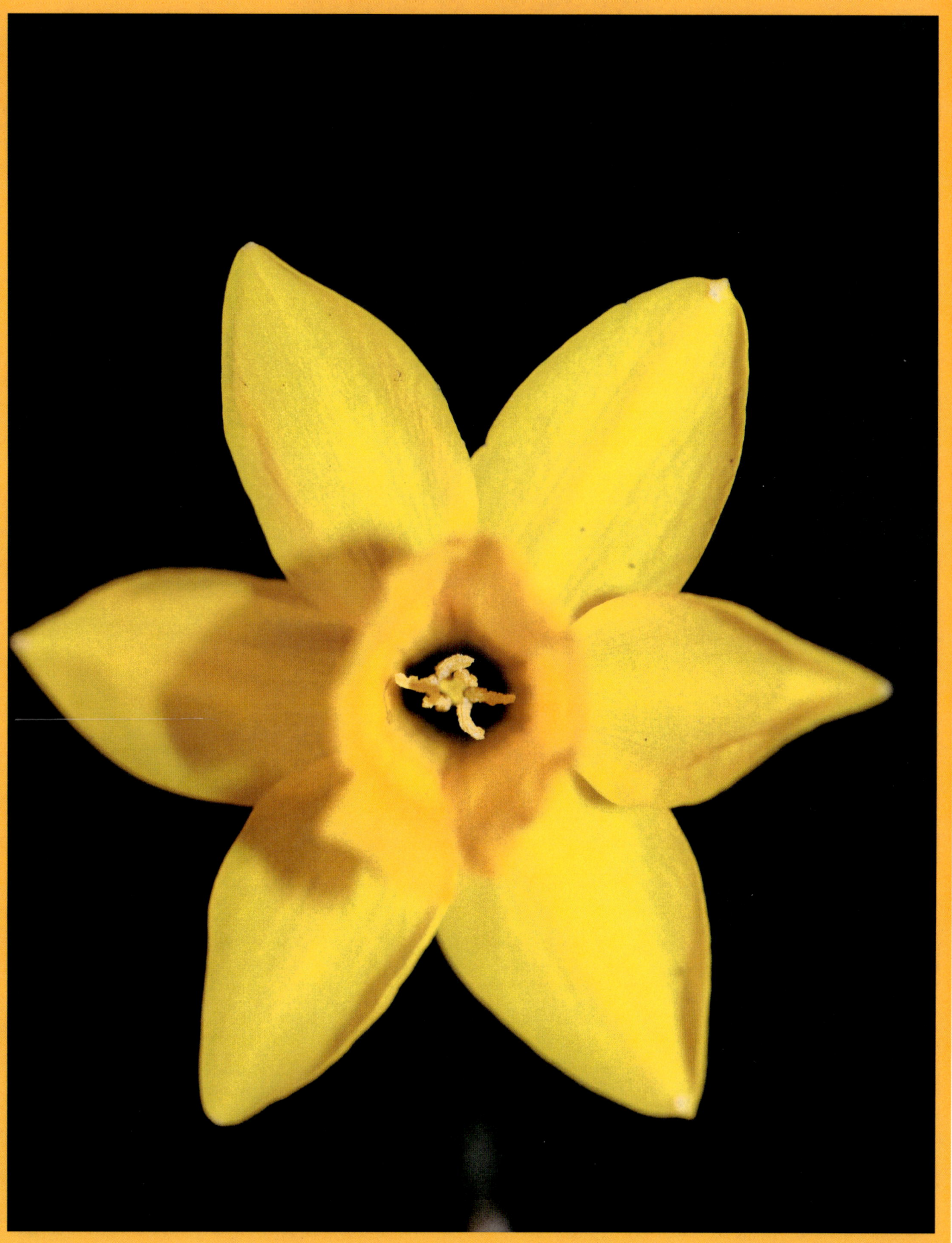

CARNATION

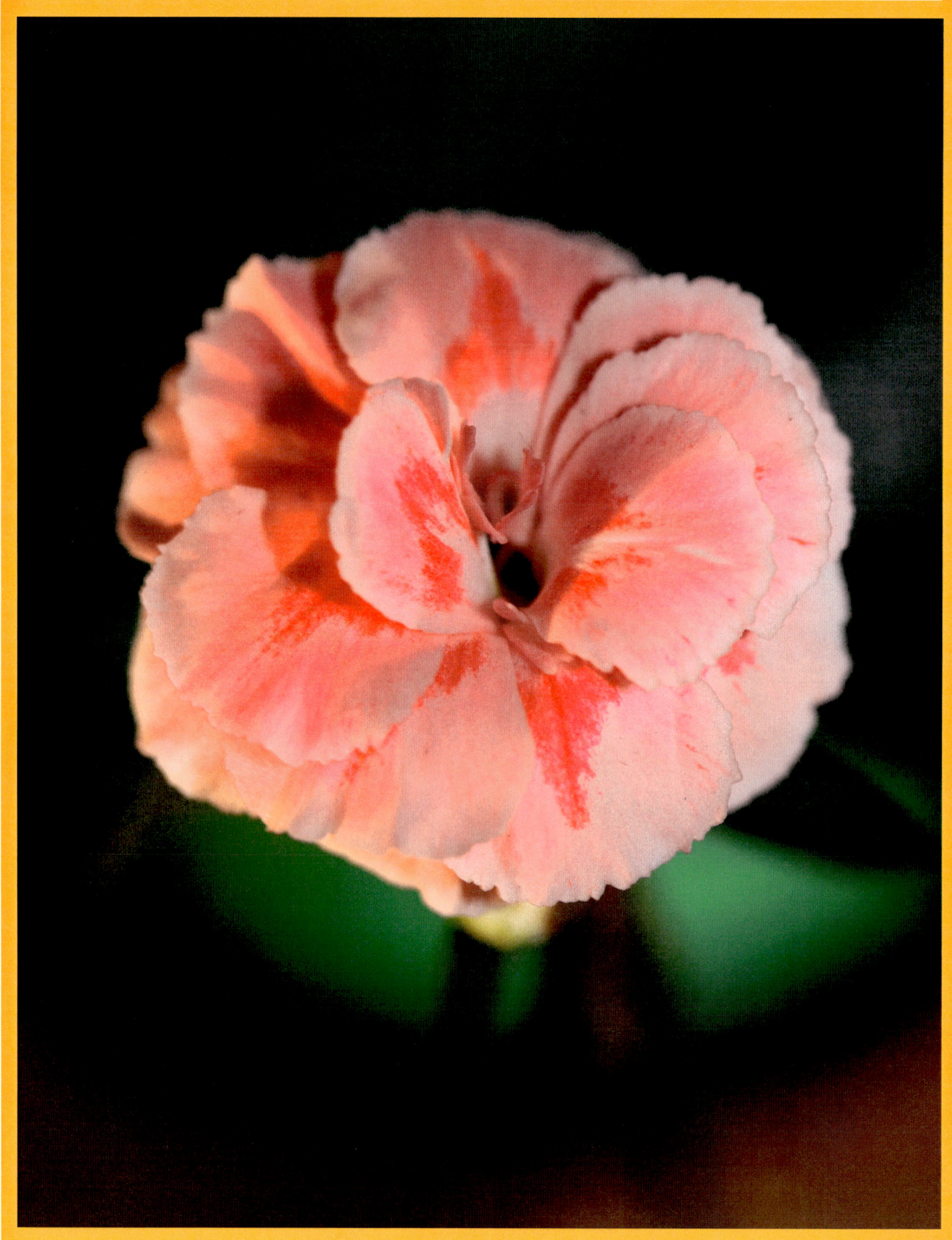

CHAMOMILE

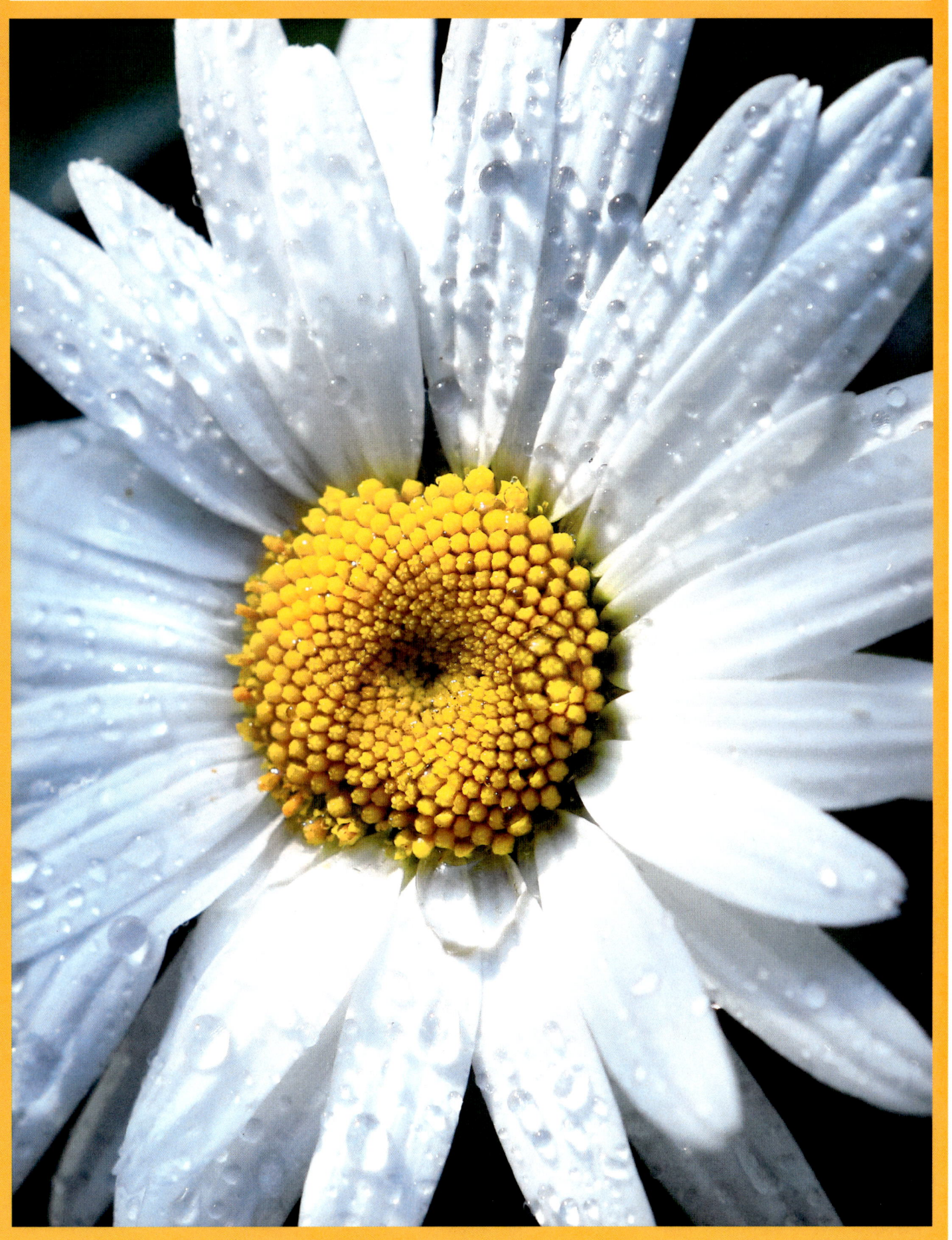

CHERRY BLOSSOM

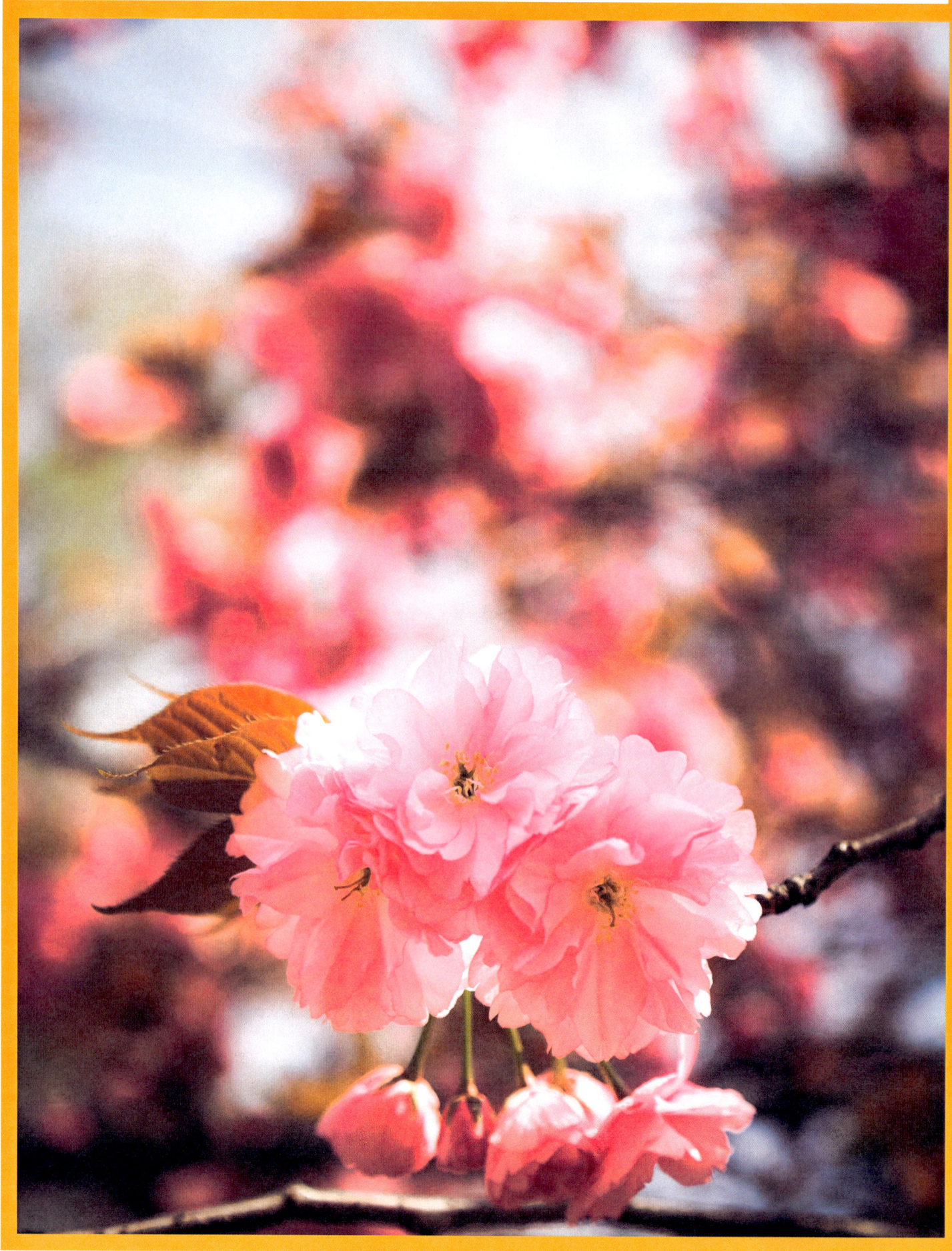

COLUMBINE

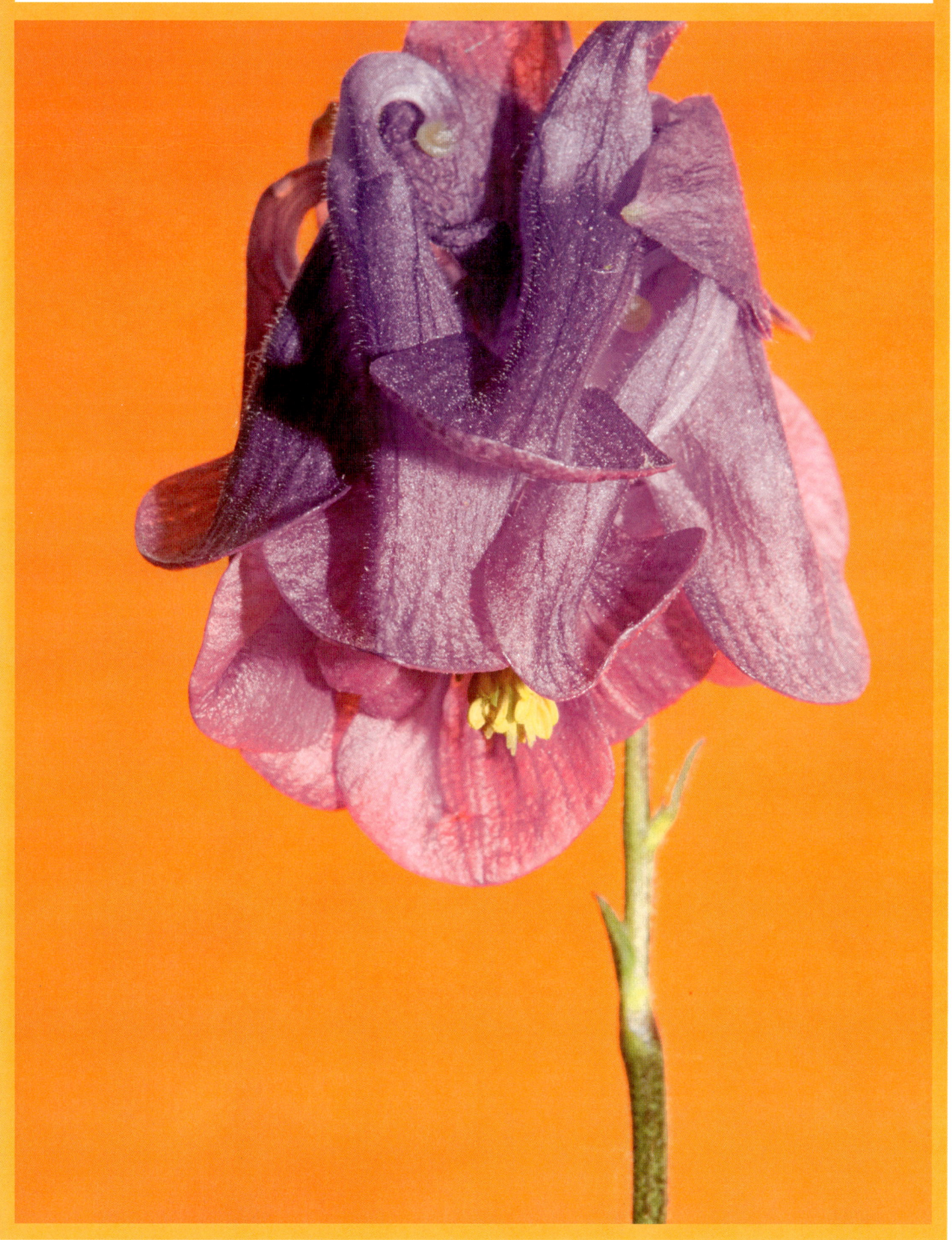

CROCUS

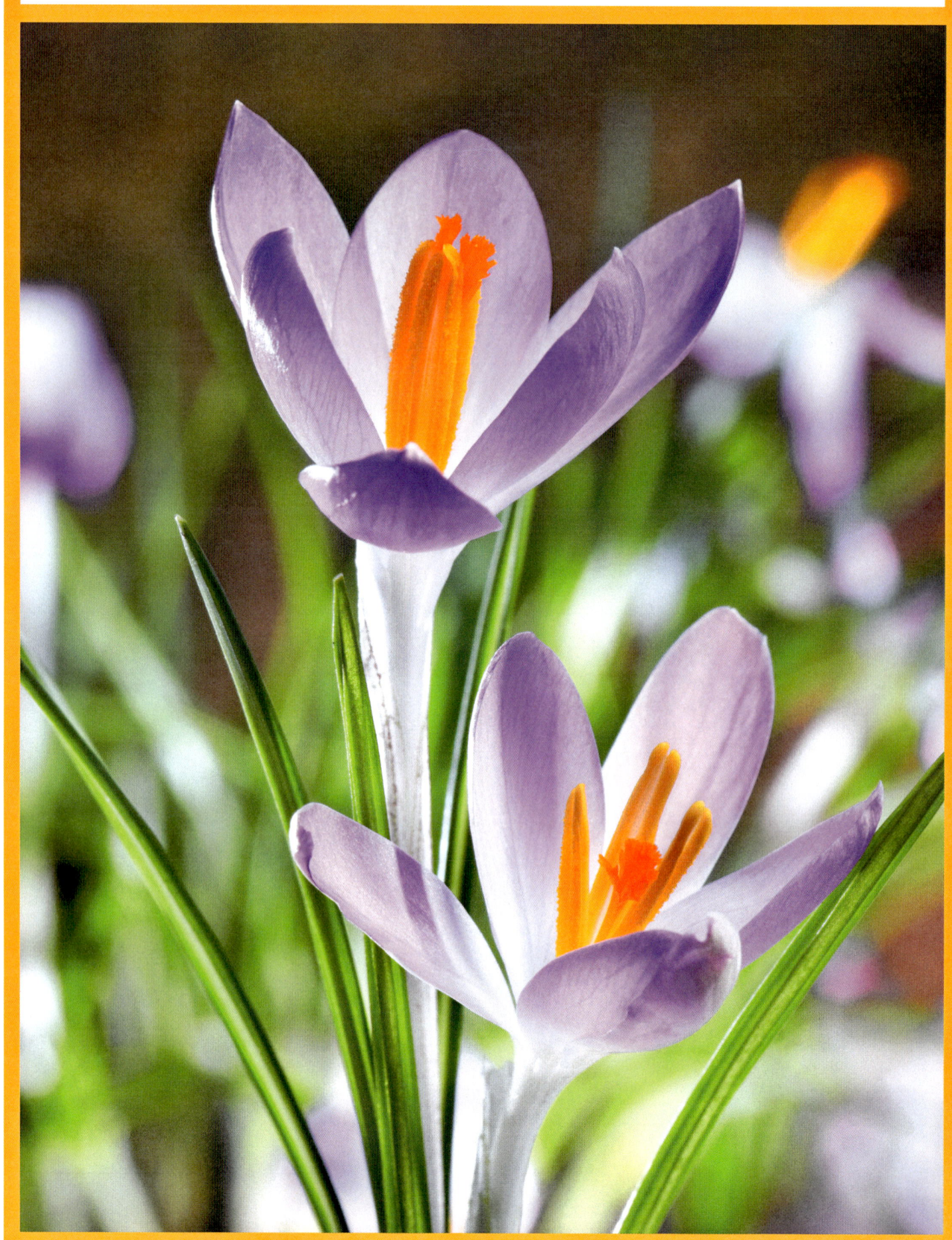

DAMASK ROSE

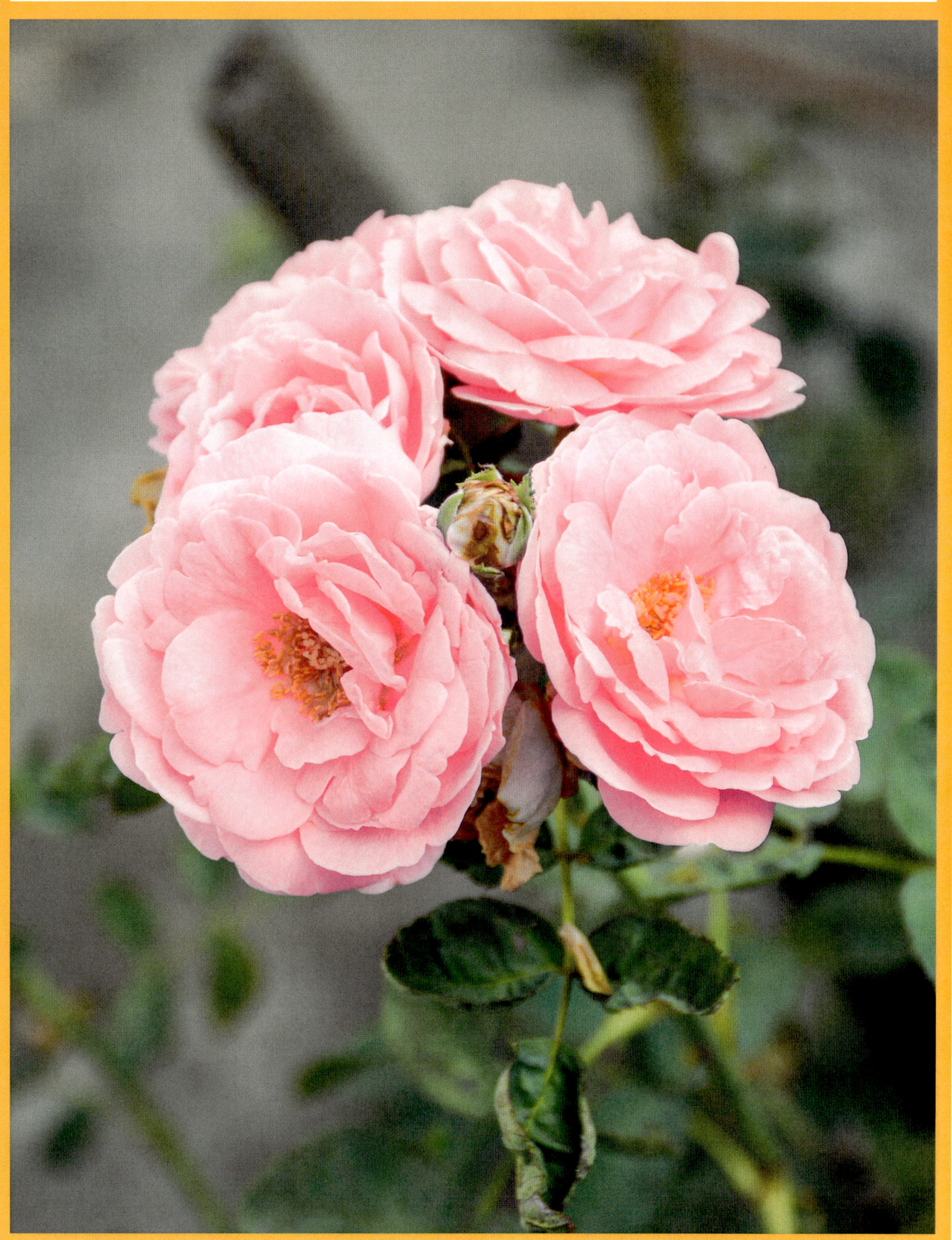

FOXGLOVE

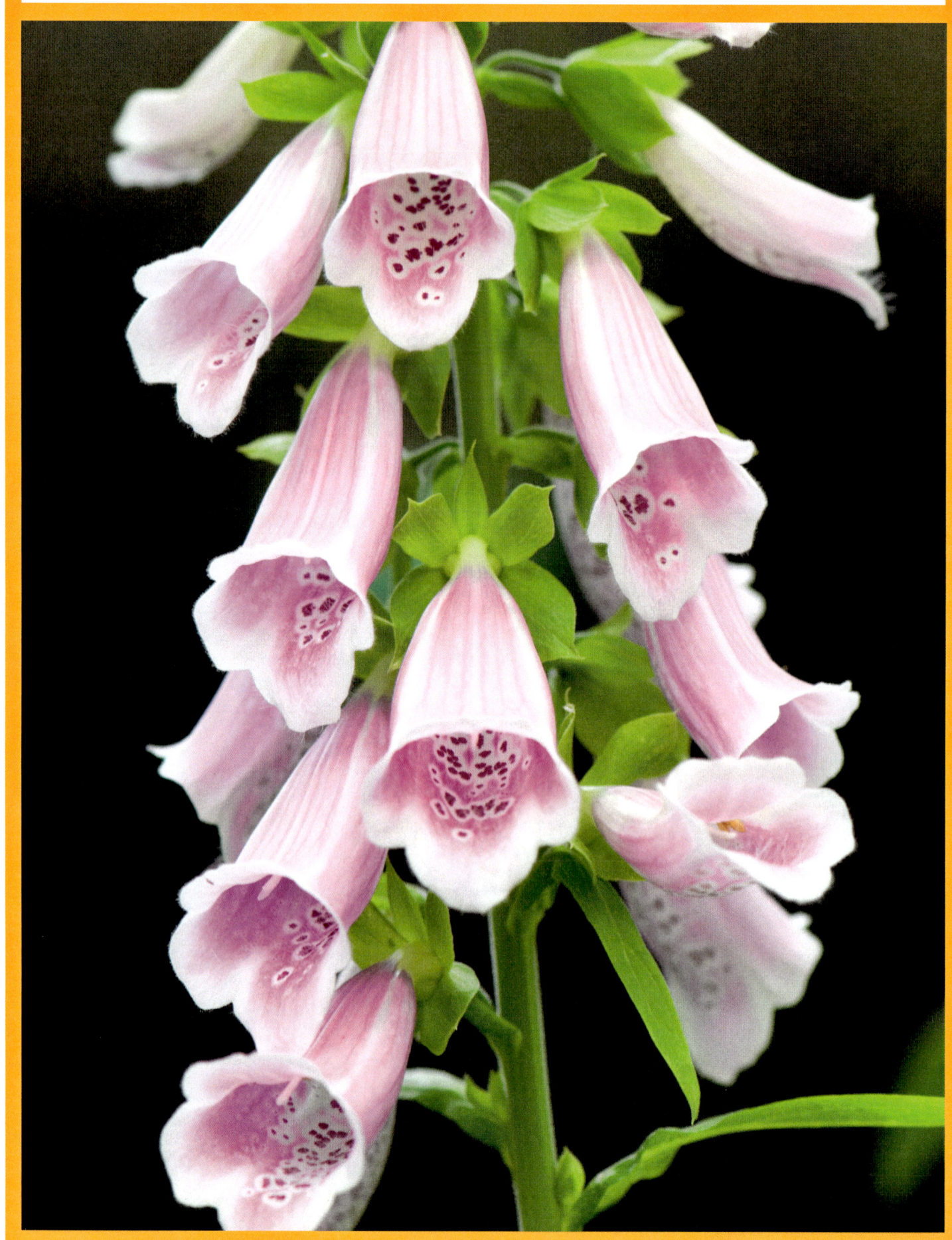

FREESIA

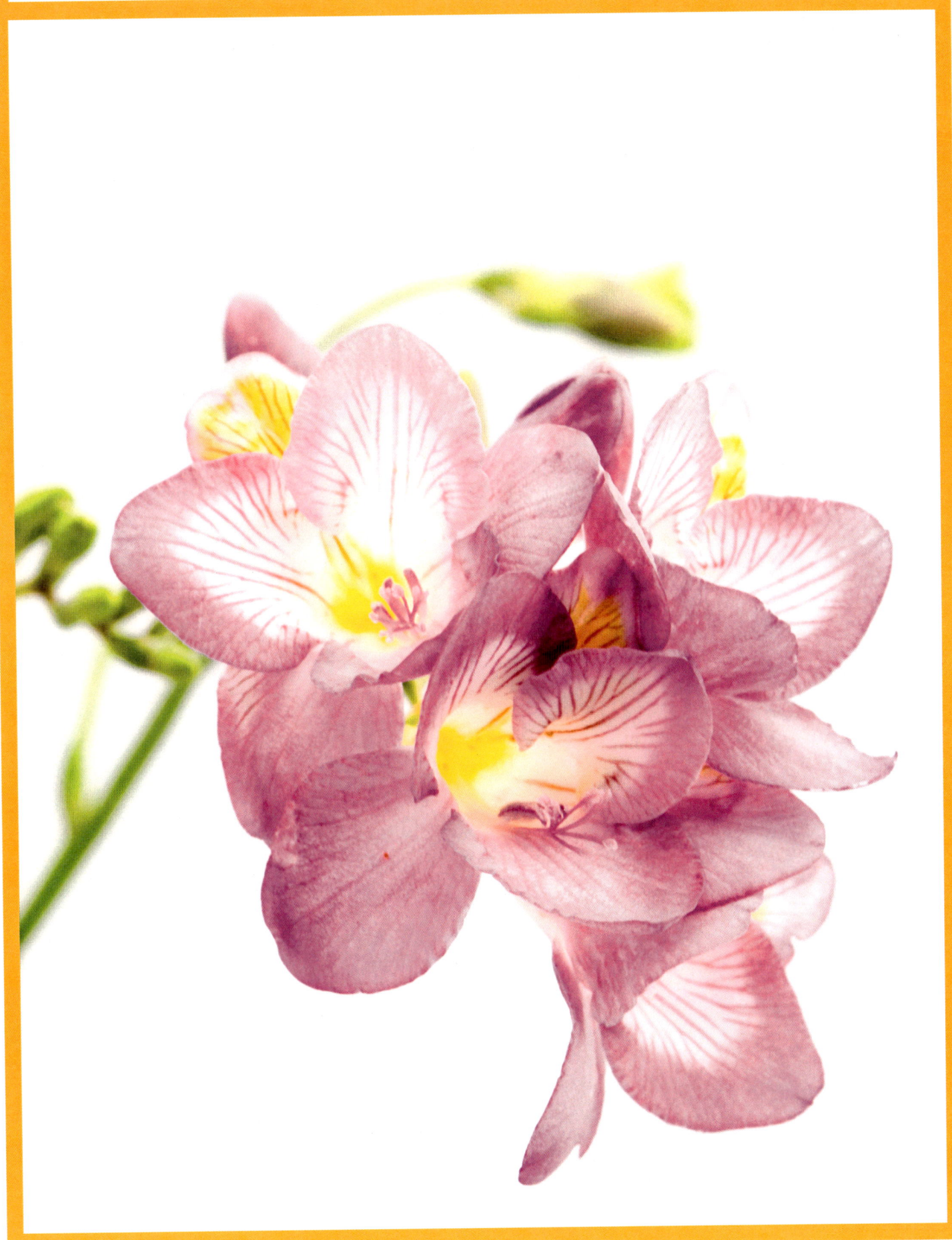

GARDENIA

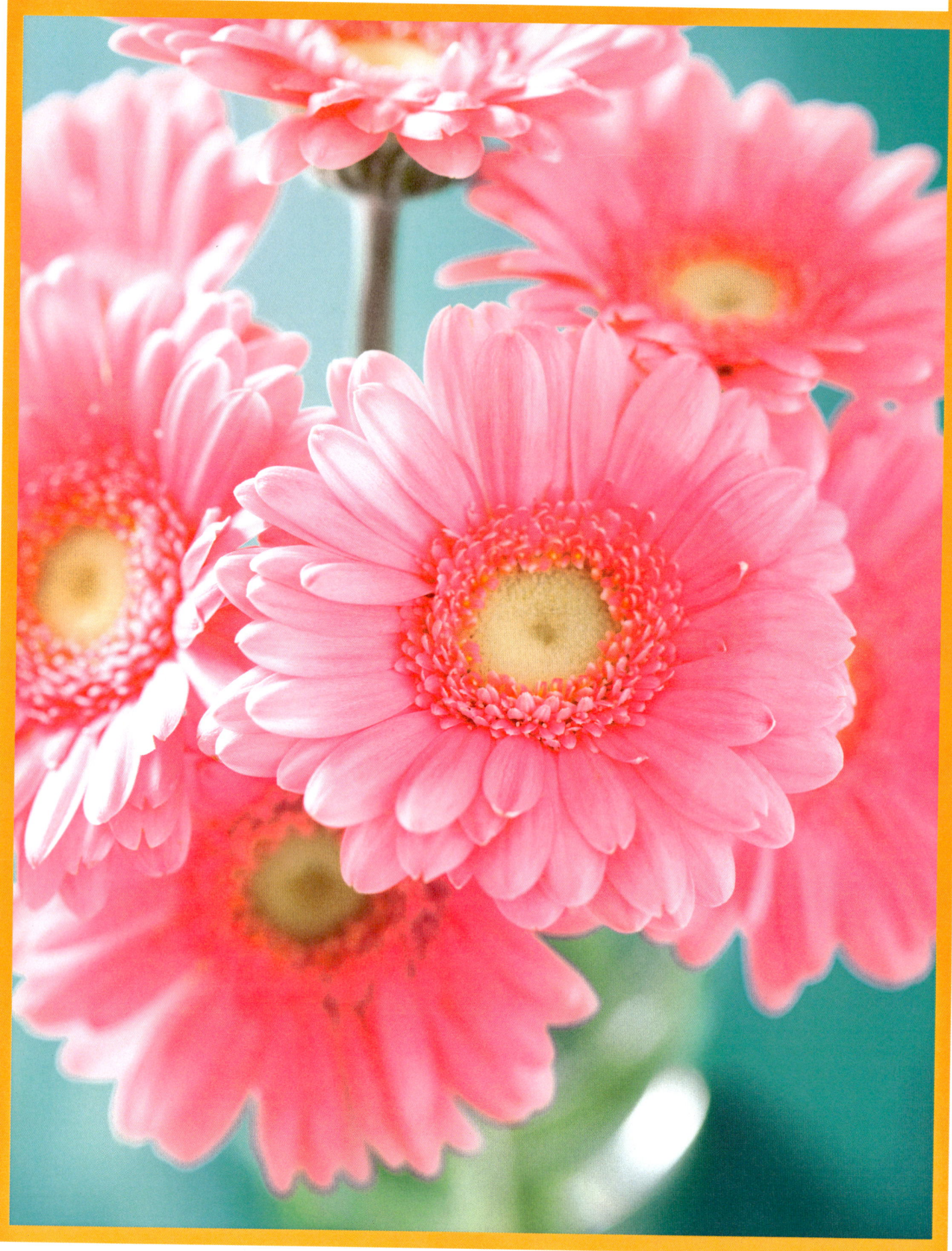

GERBERA

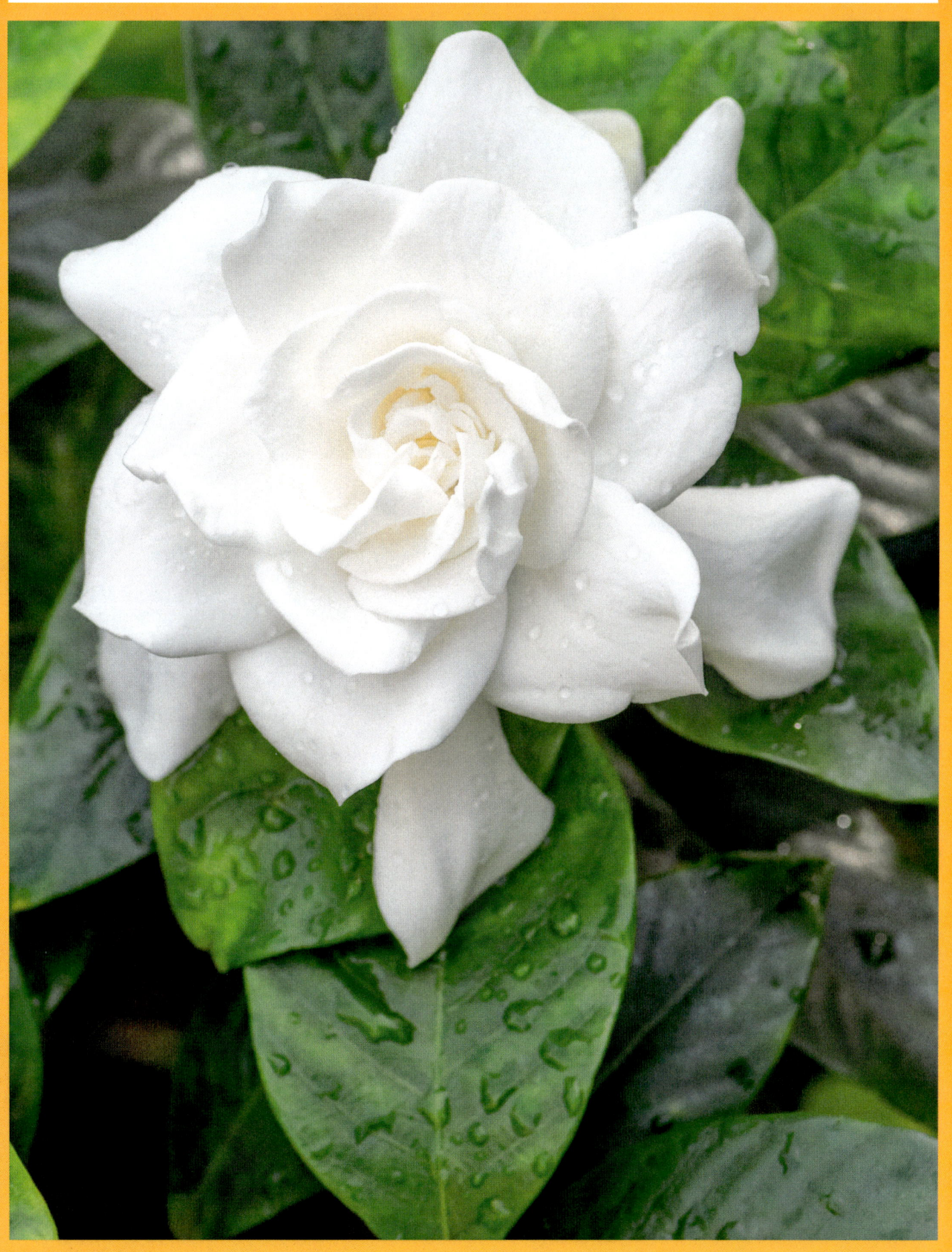

YELLOW ROSE

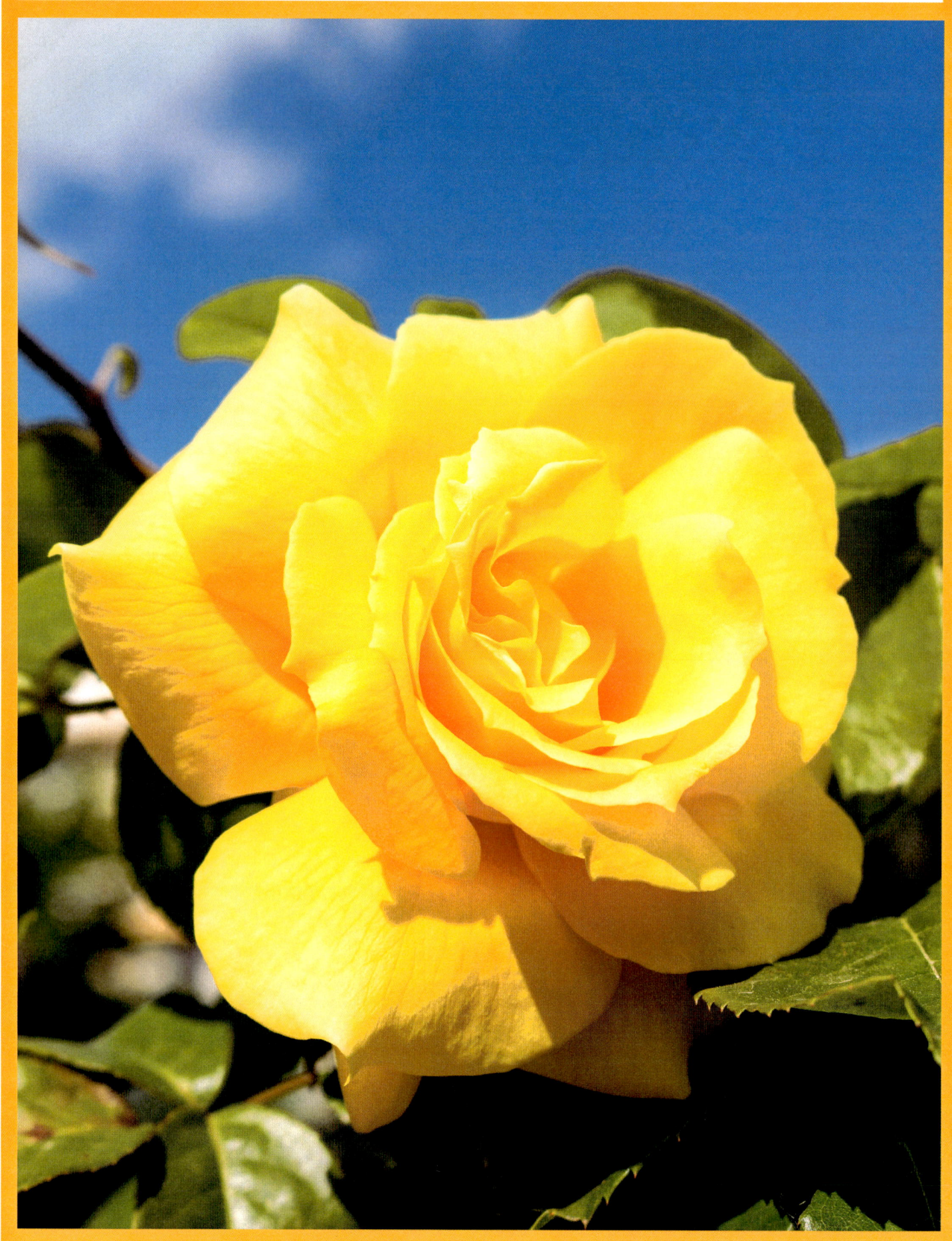

GLADIOLUS

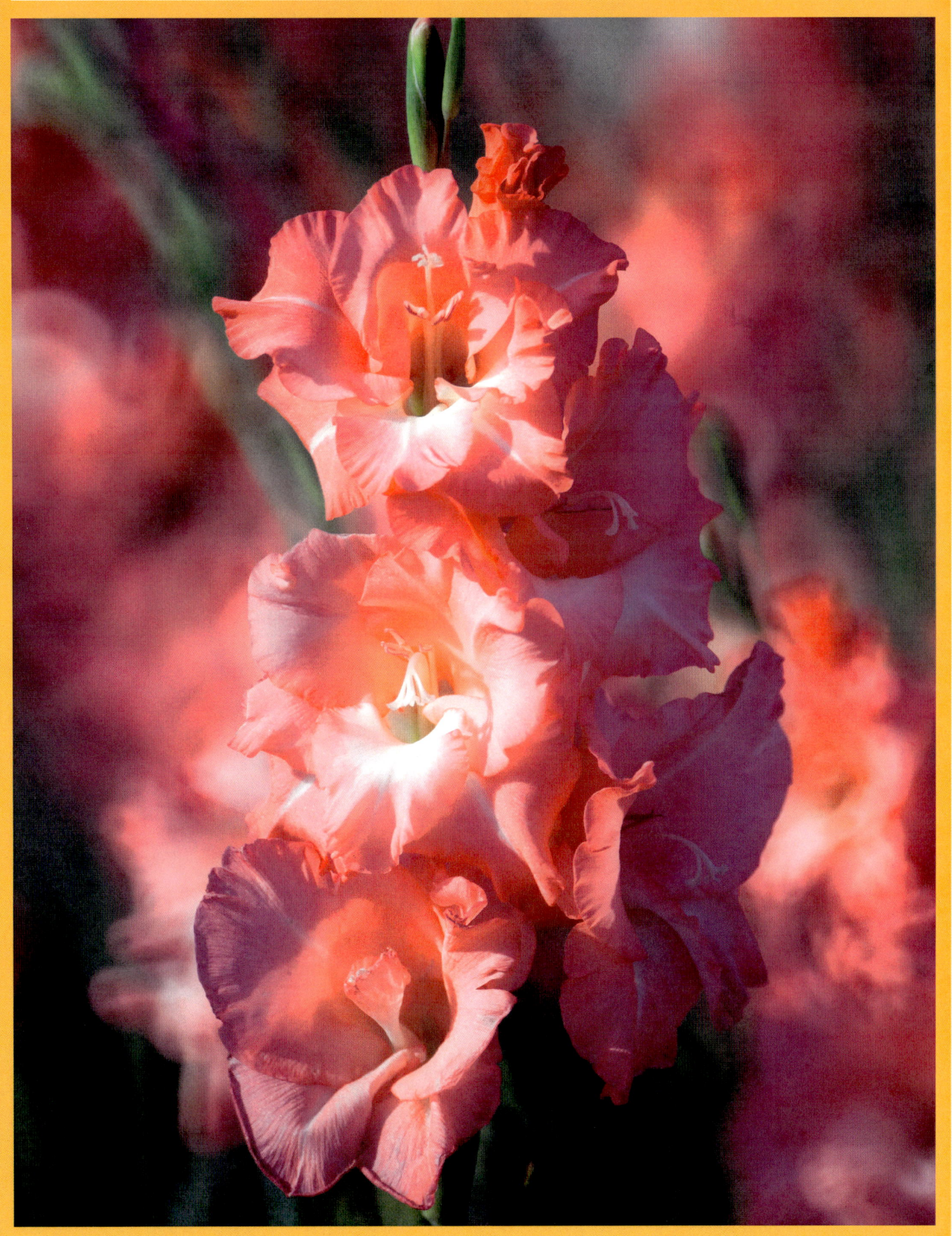

HYDRANGEA

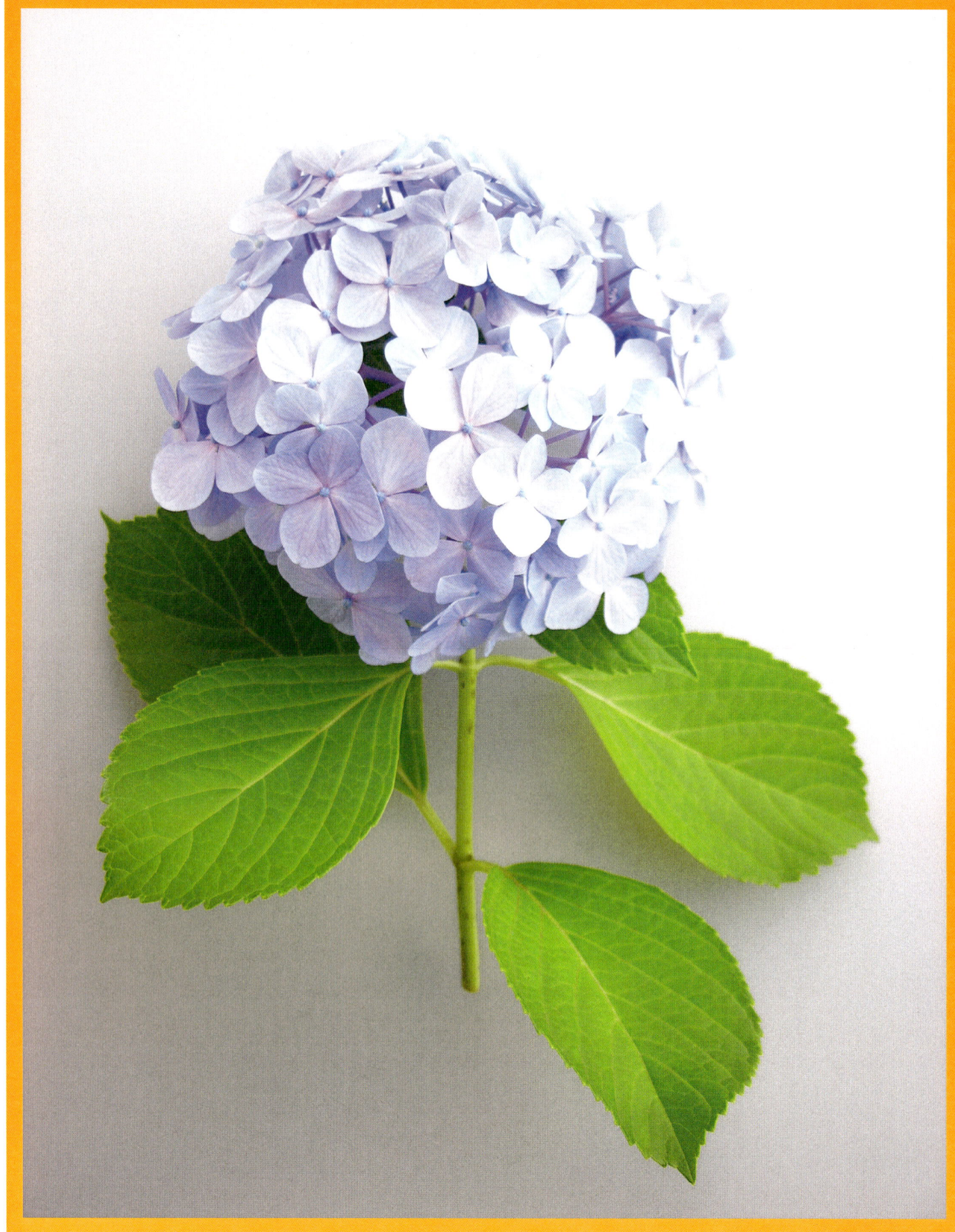

INDIGO FLOWER

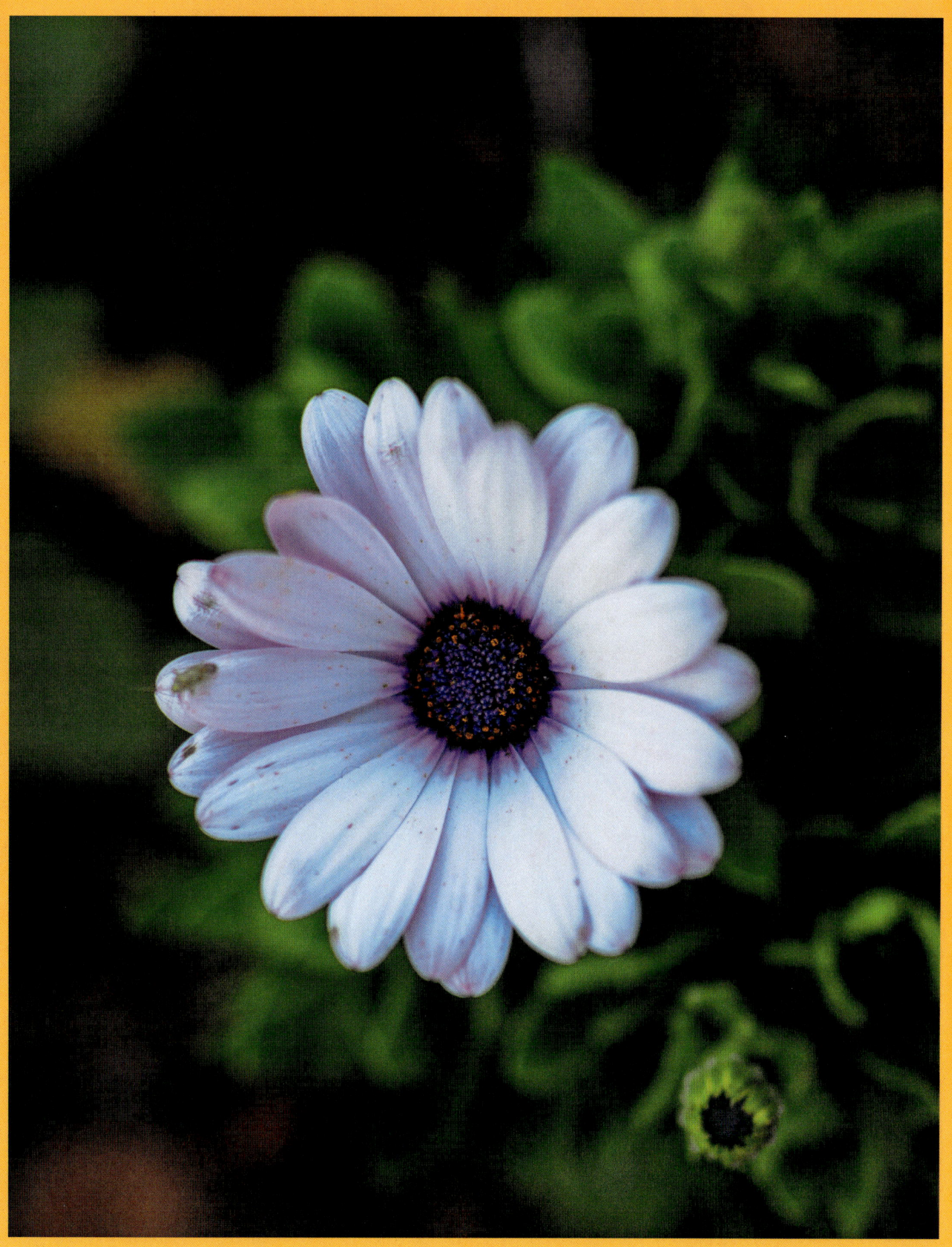

LANTANAS

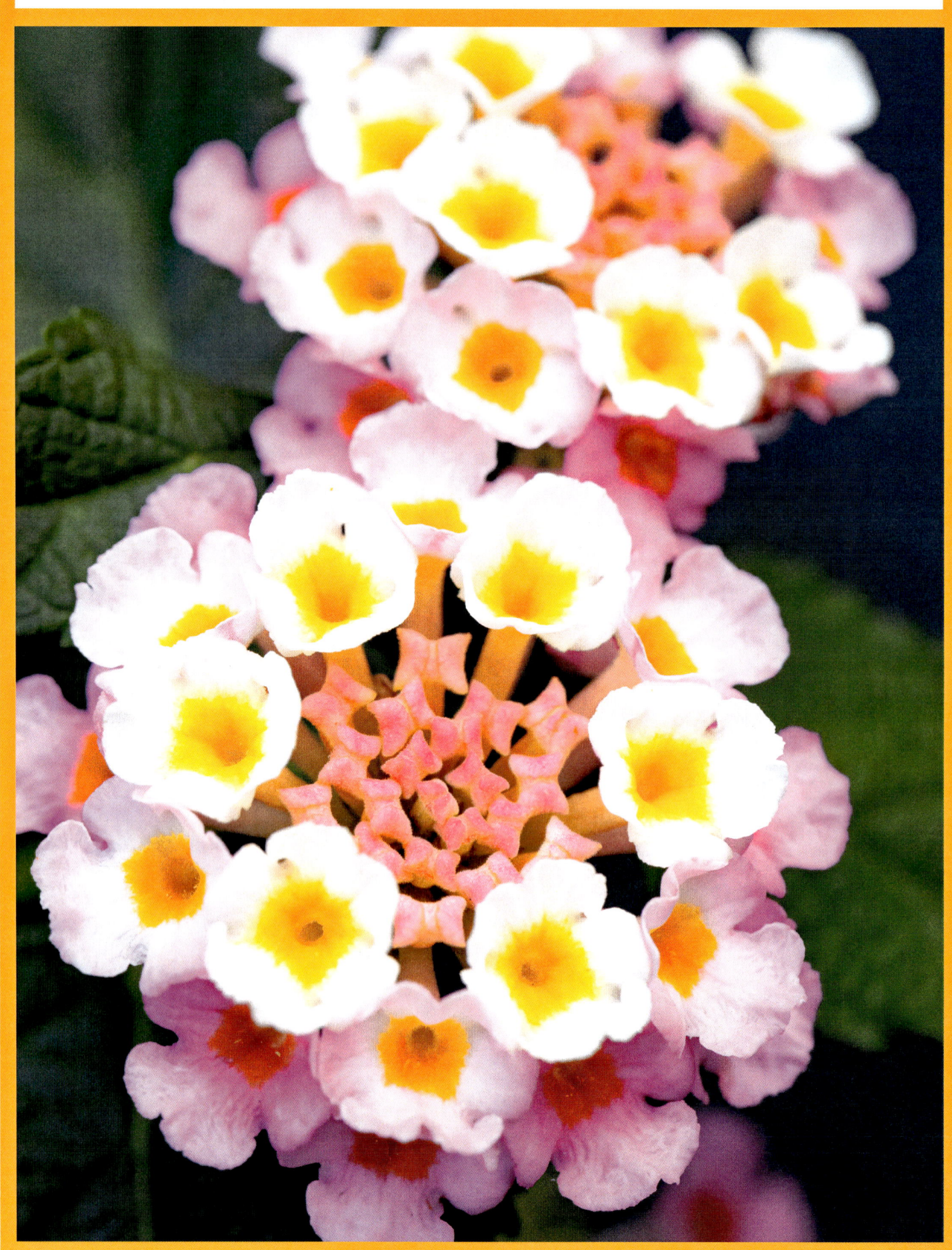

LEOPARD LILY

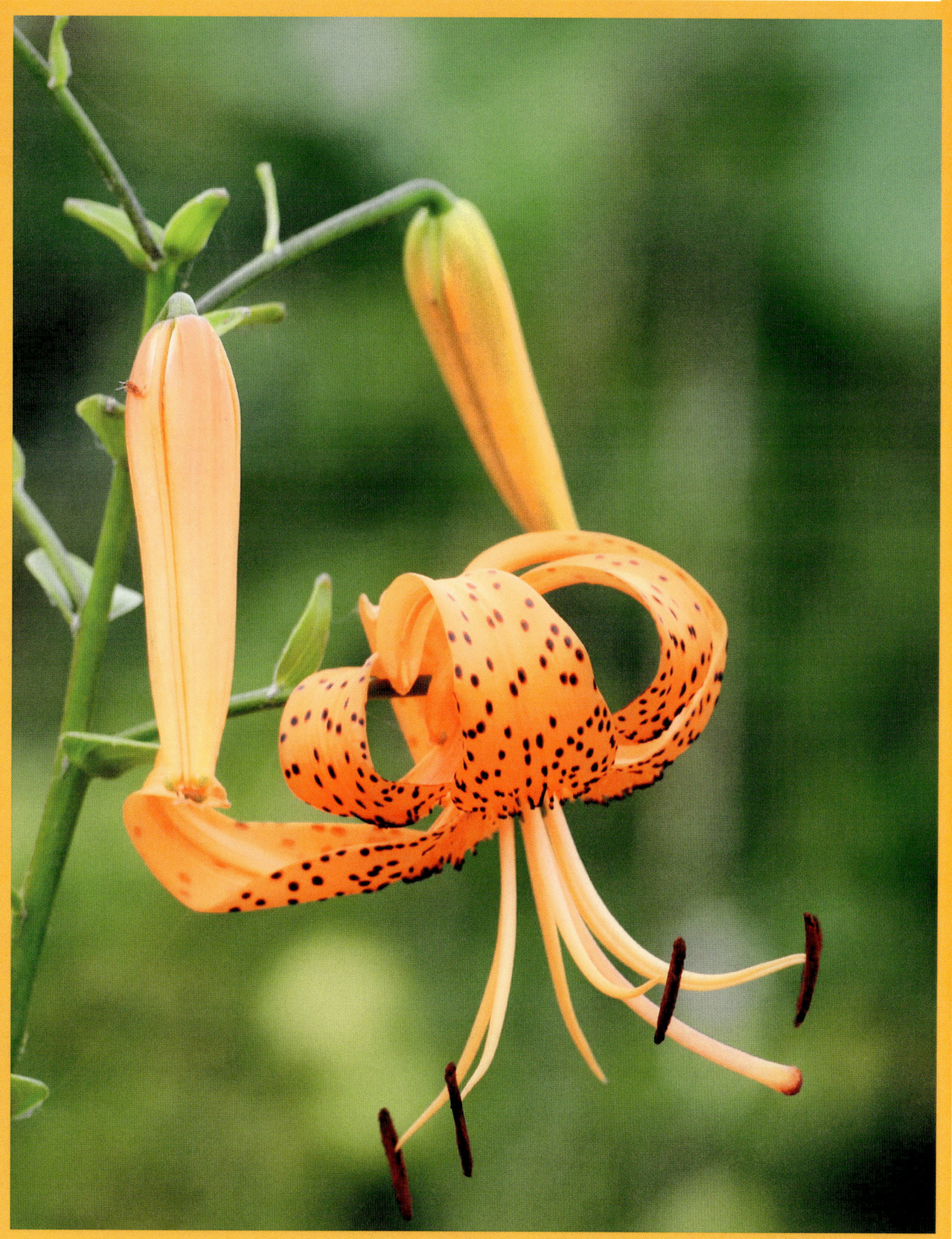

LILAC

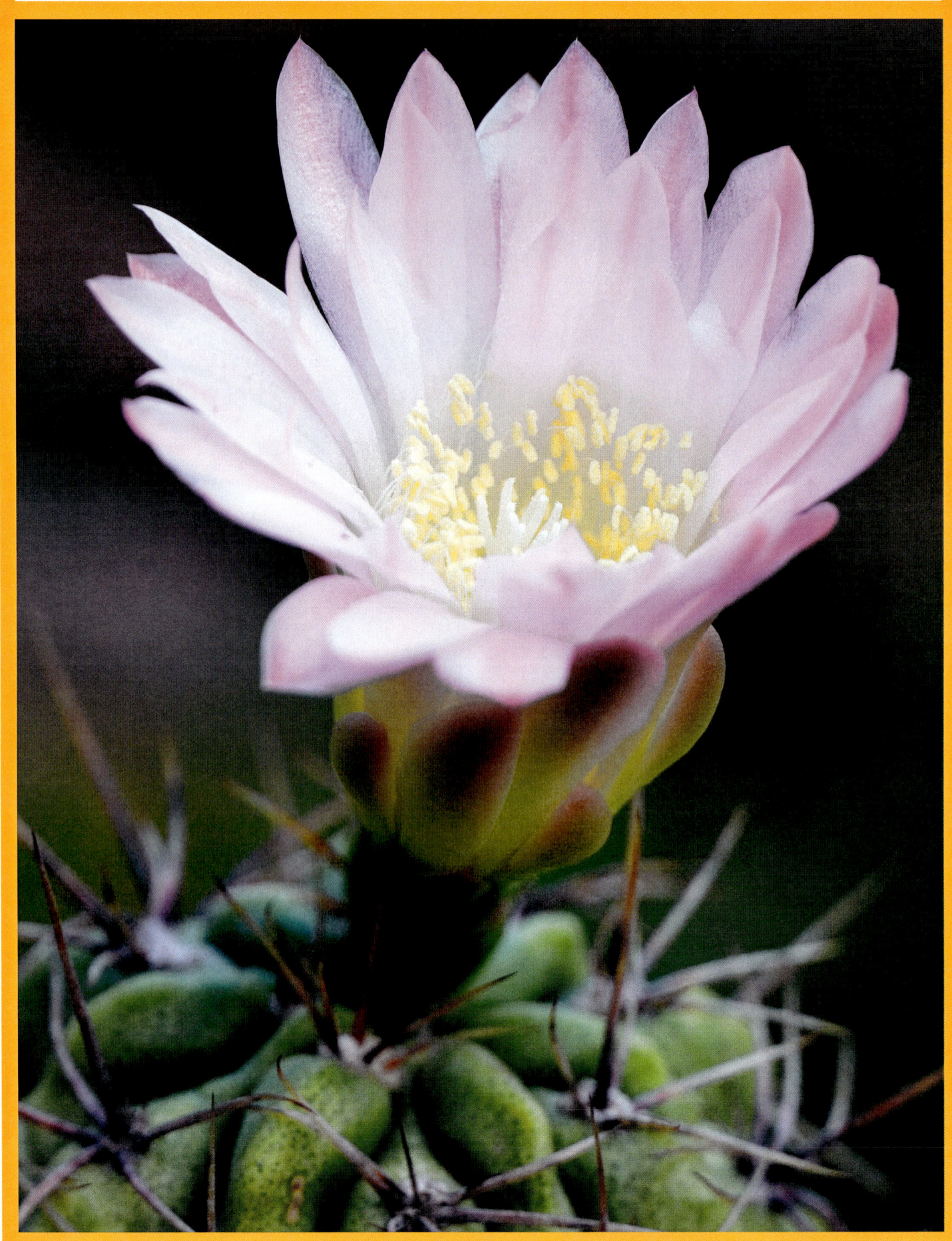

RED LILY

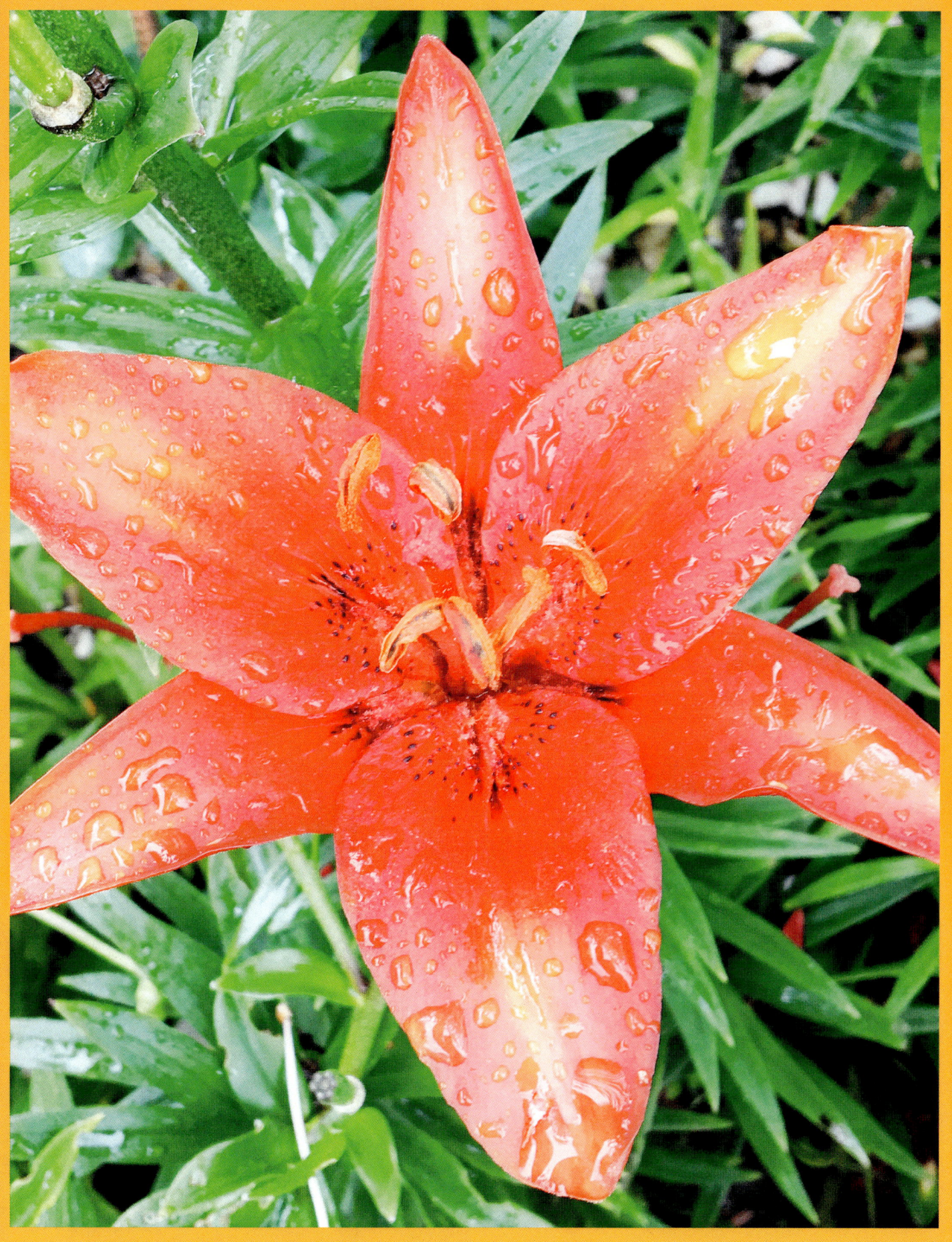

LIVERWORT FLOWER

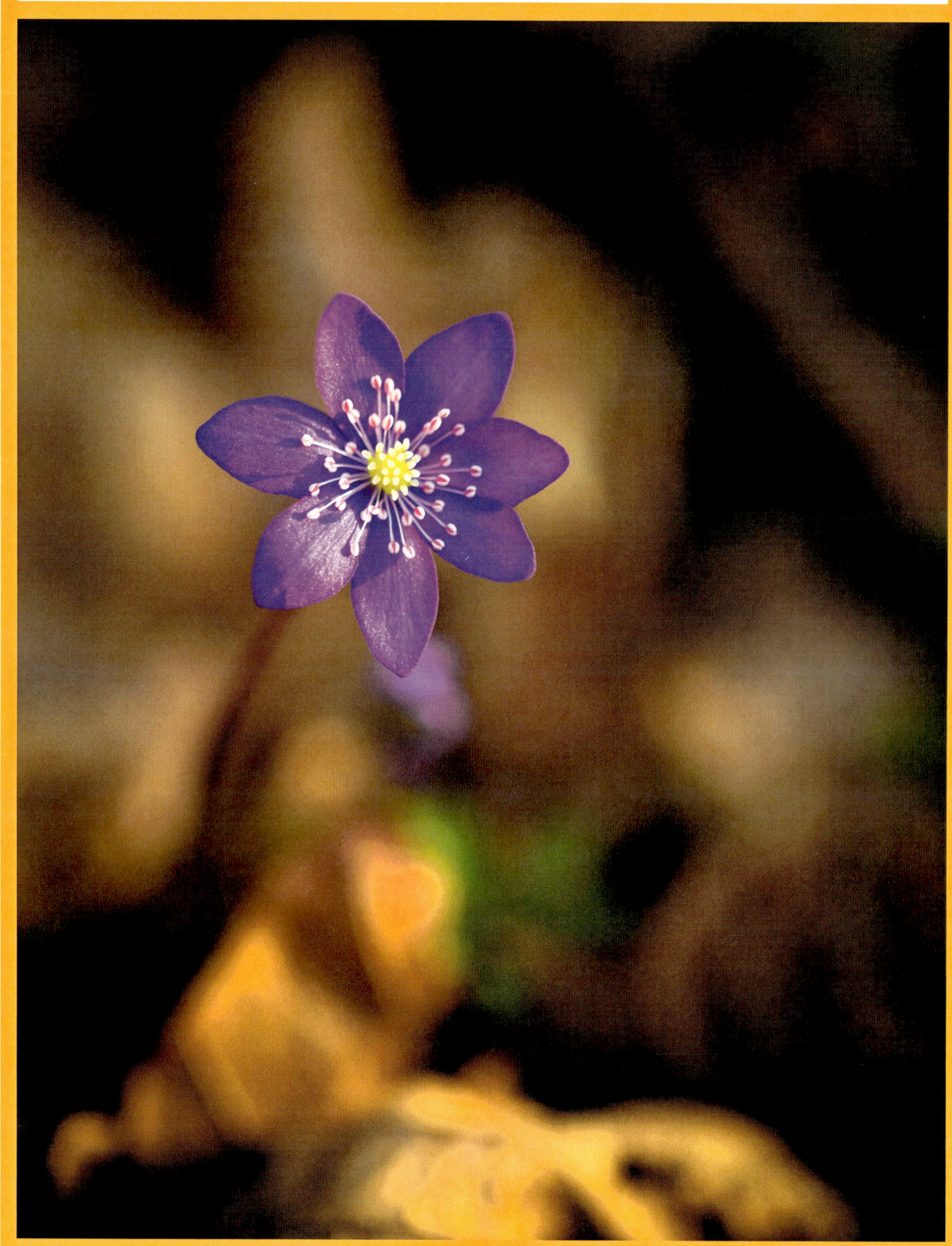

LOTUS

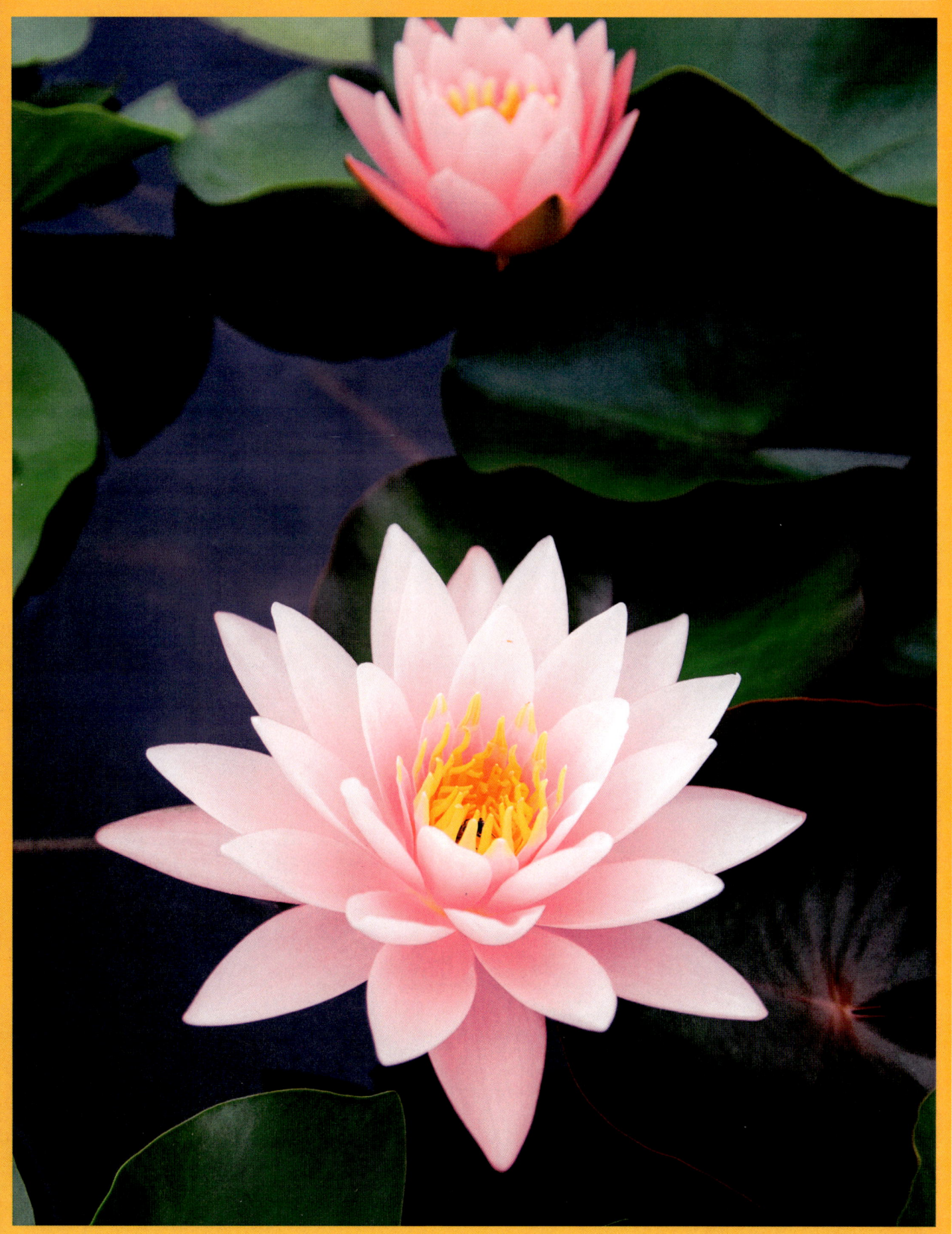

MAGNOLIA

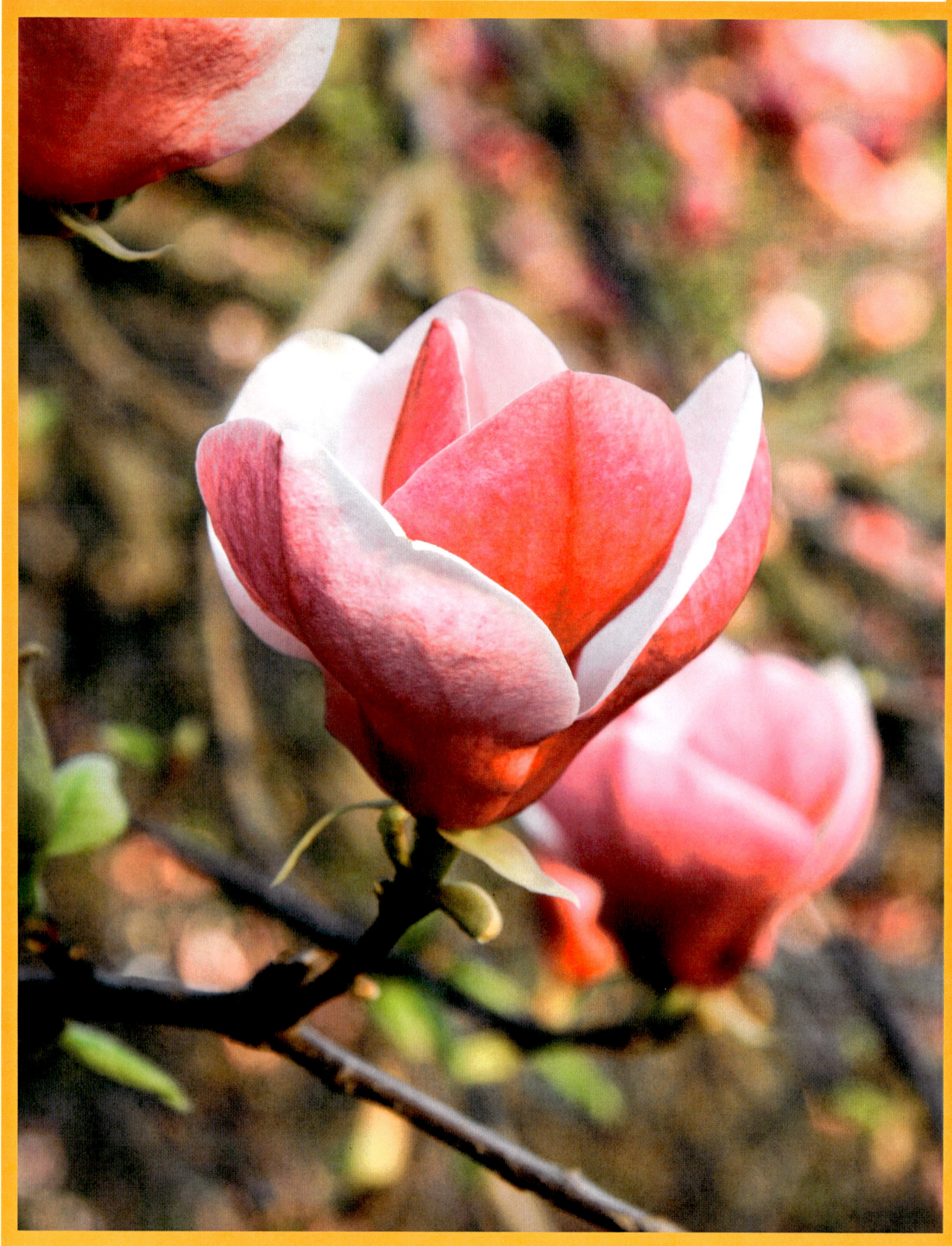

MARIGOLD

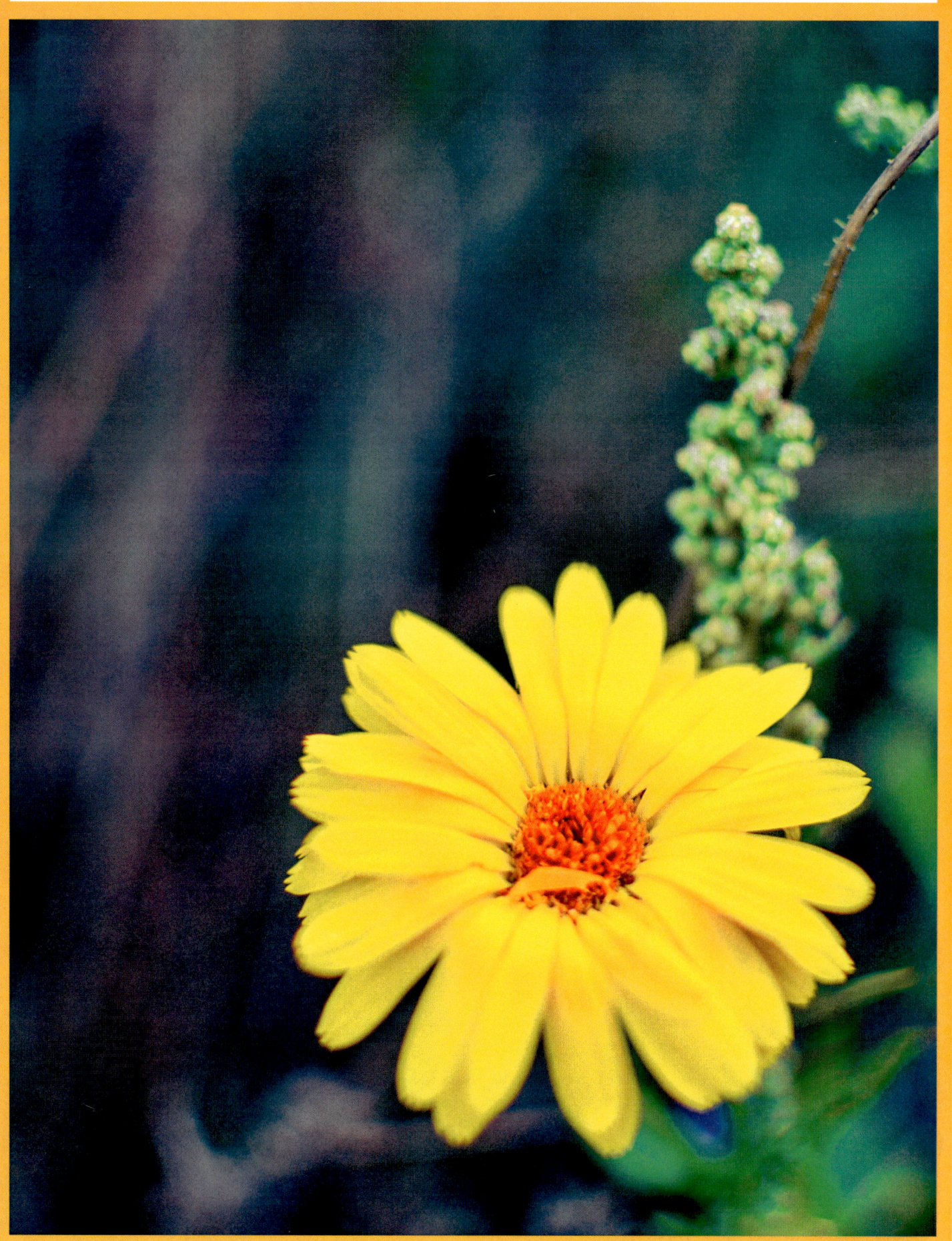

ORANGE ZINNIA

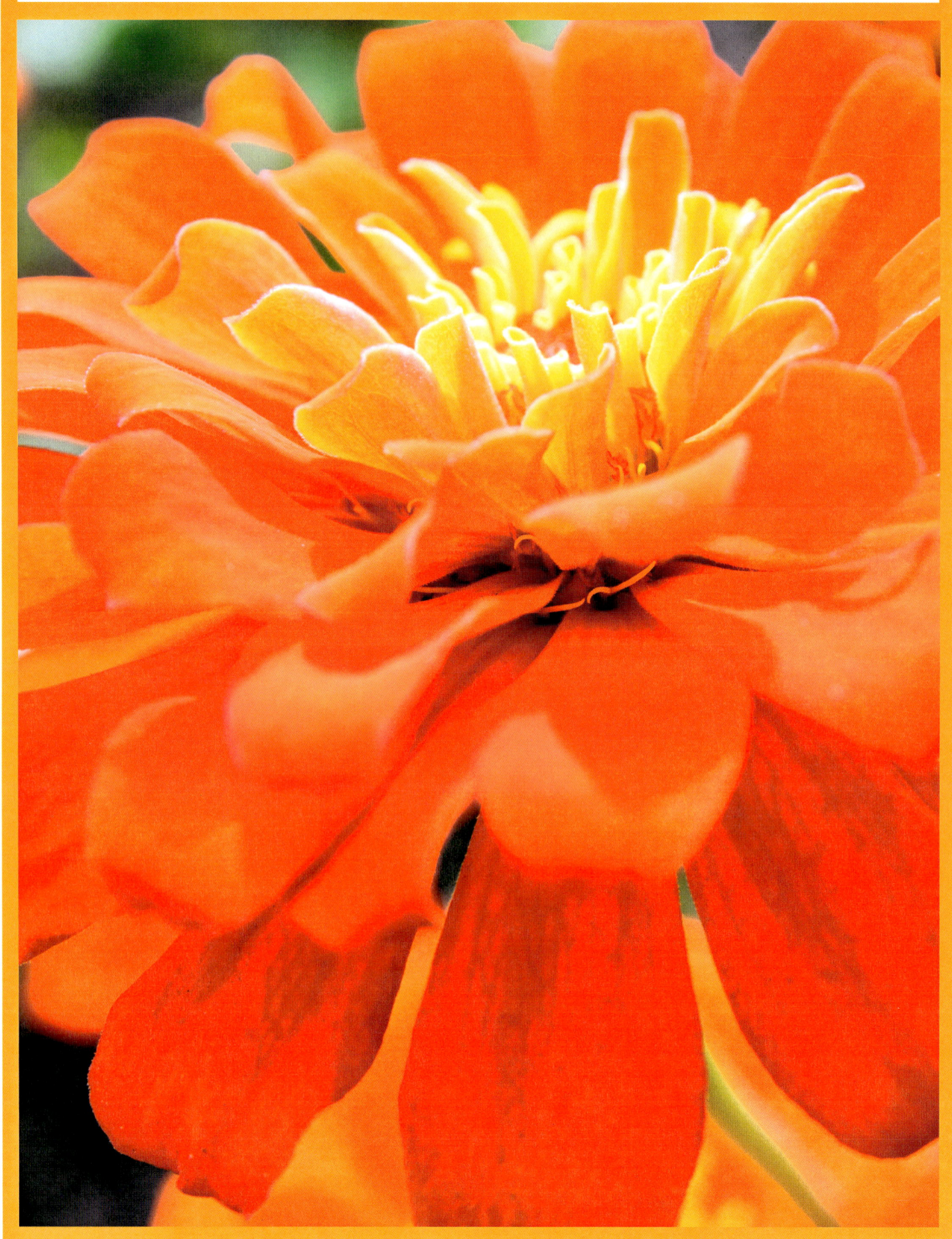

PASSION FLOWER

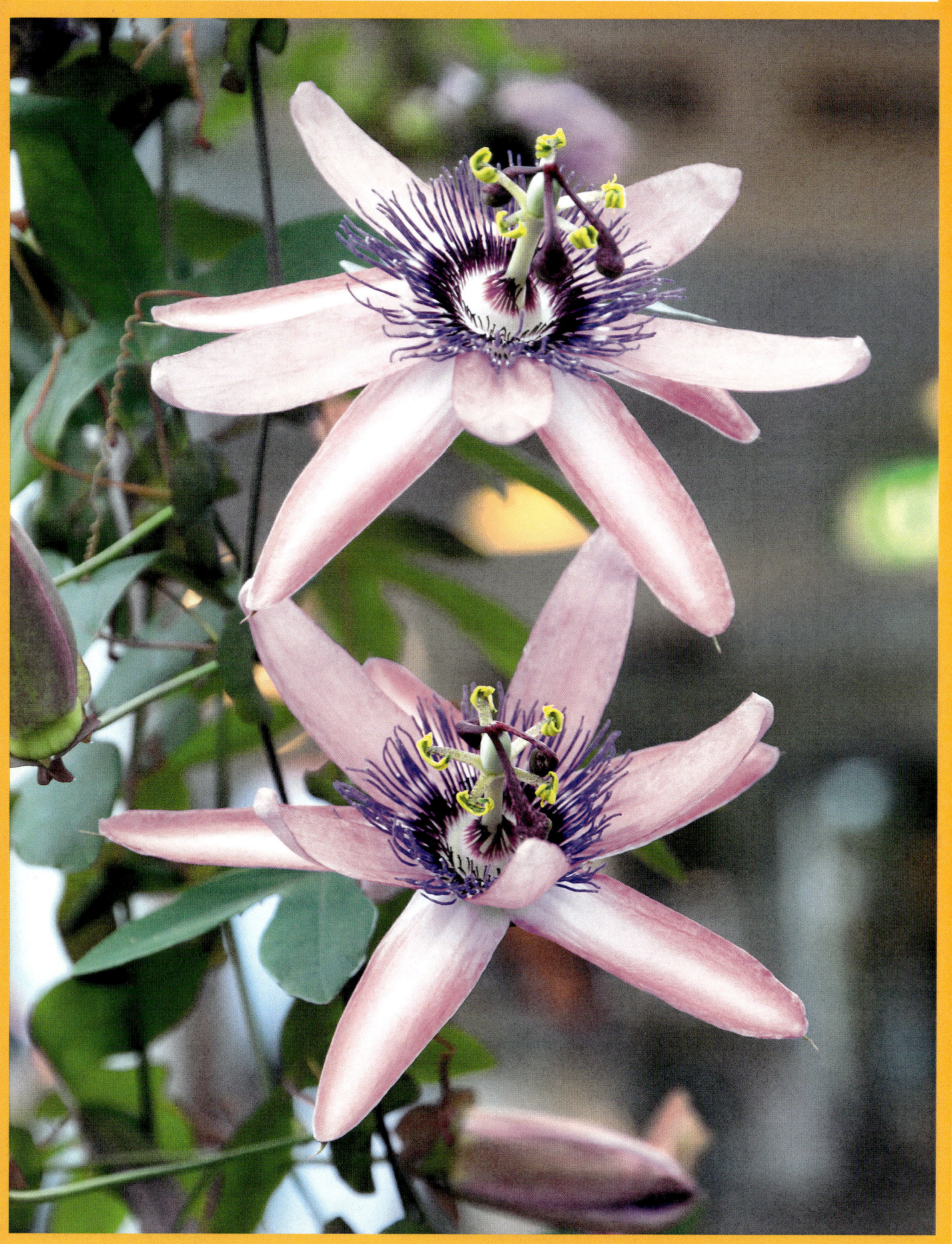

PEONY

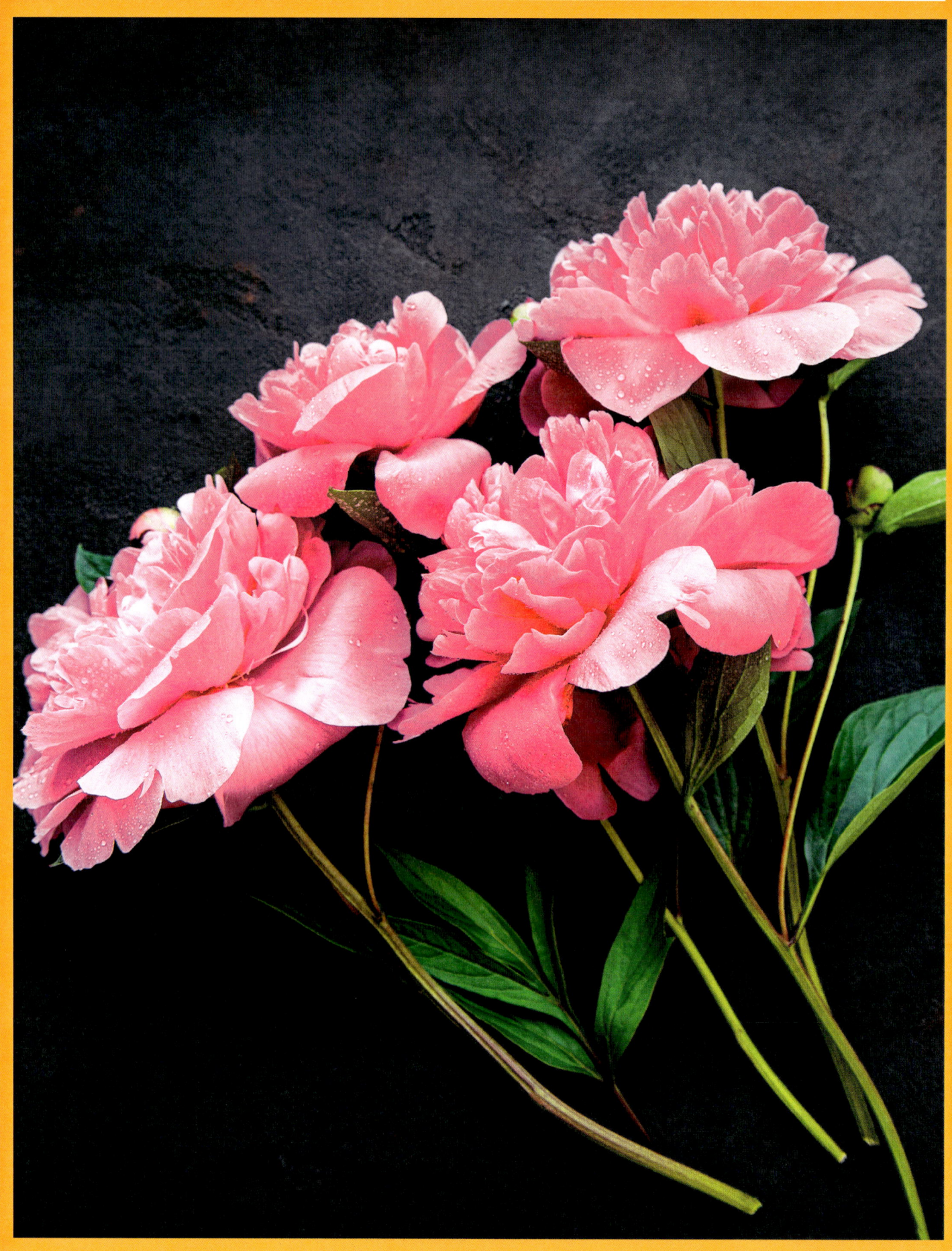

POPPY FLOWER

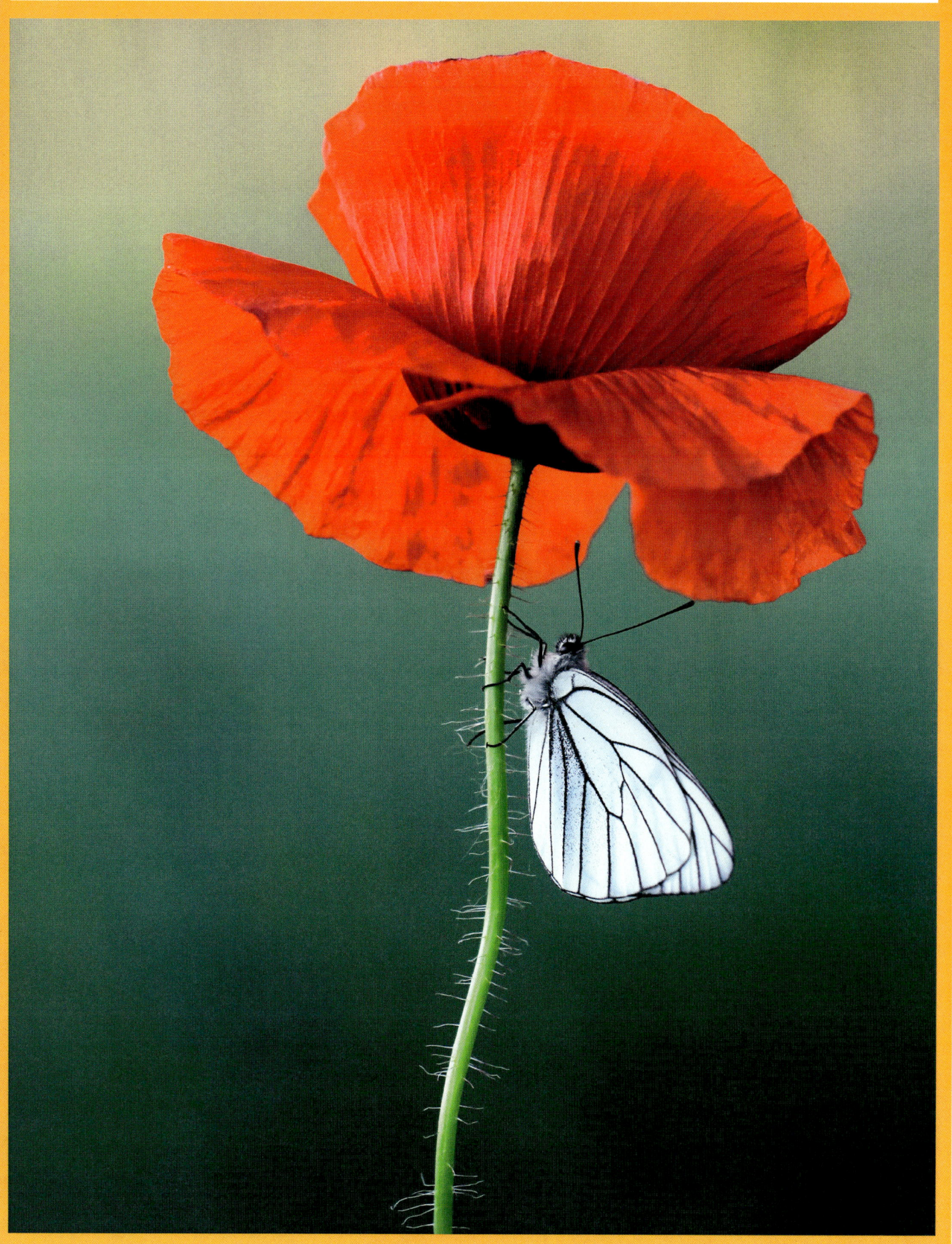

PROTEA FLOWER

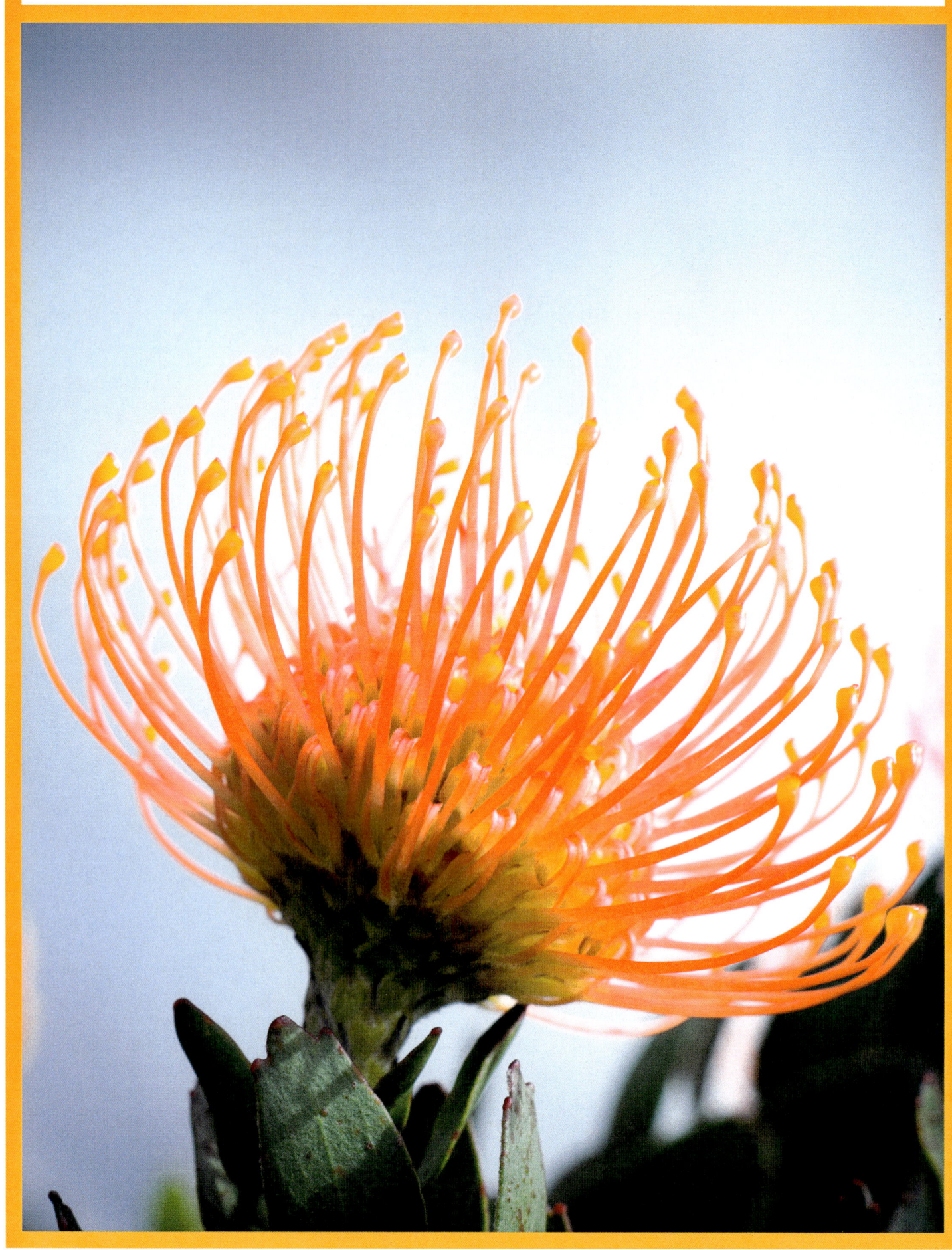

RANUNCULUS

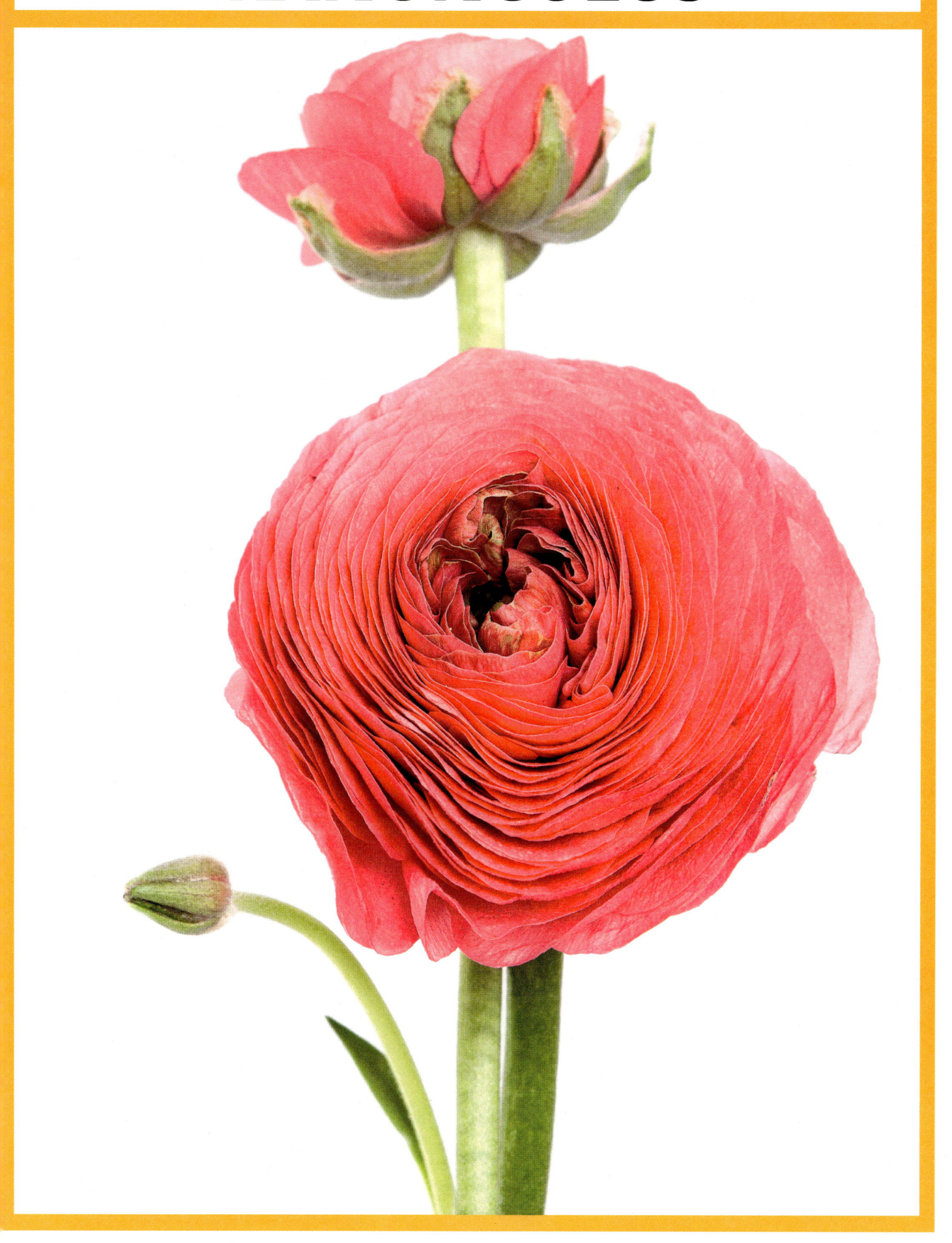

RED AMARYLLIS

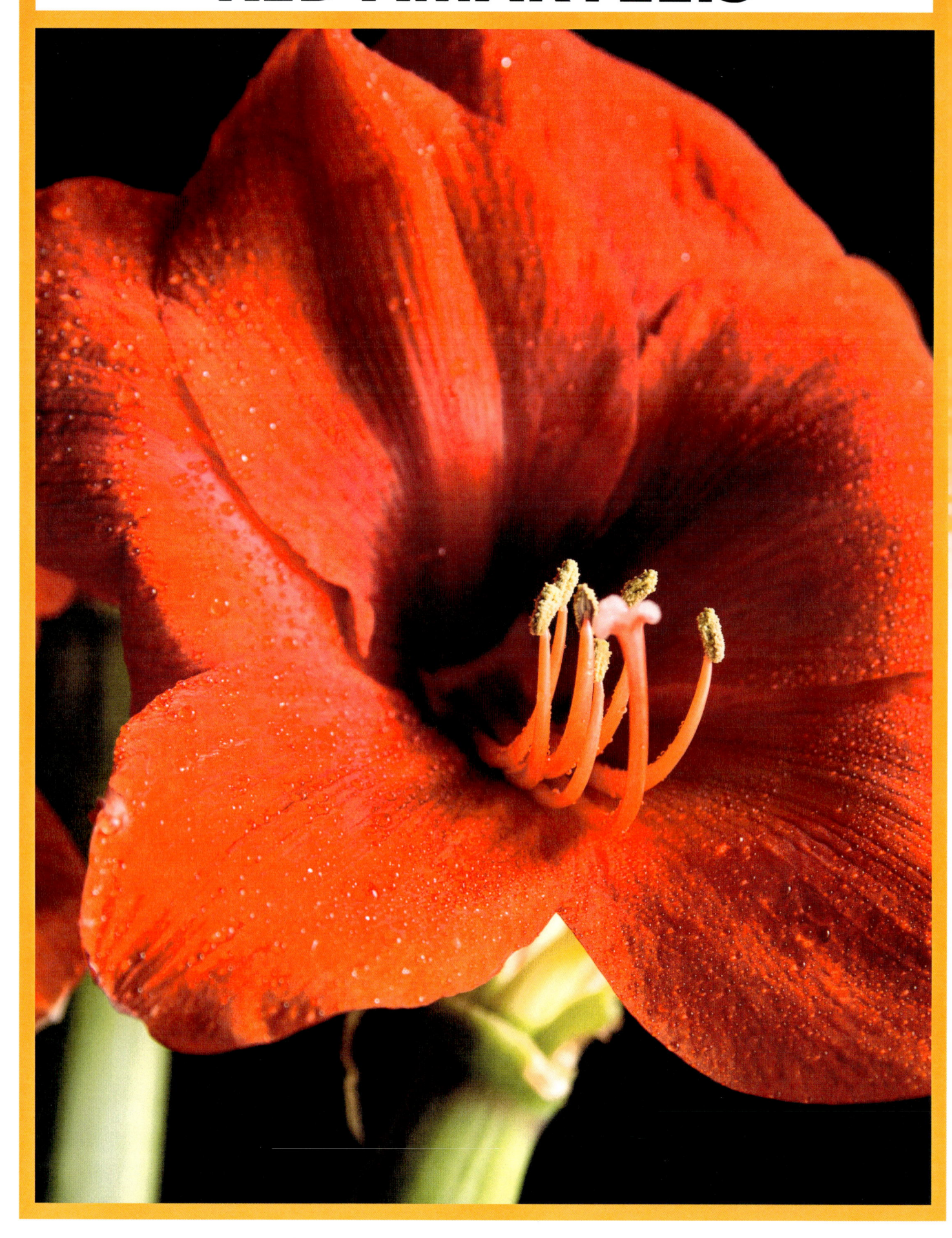

RED MALLOW

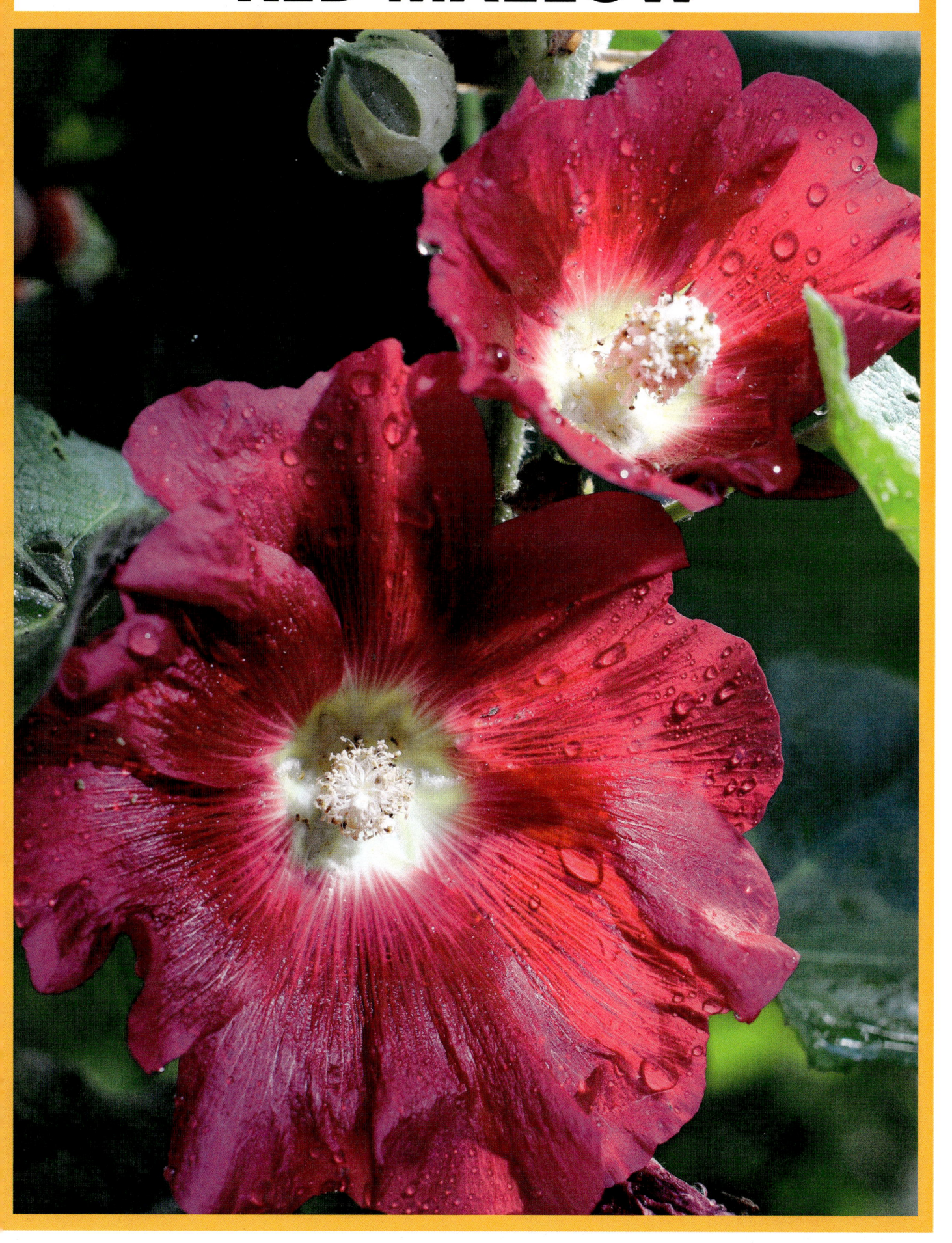

RED ROSE

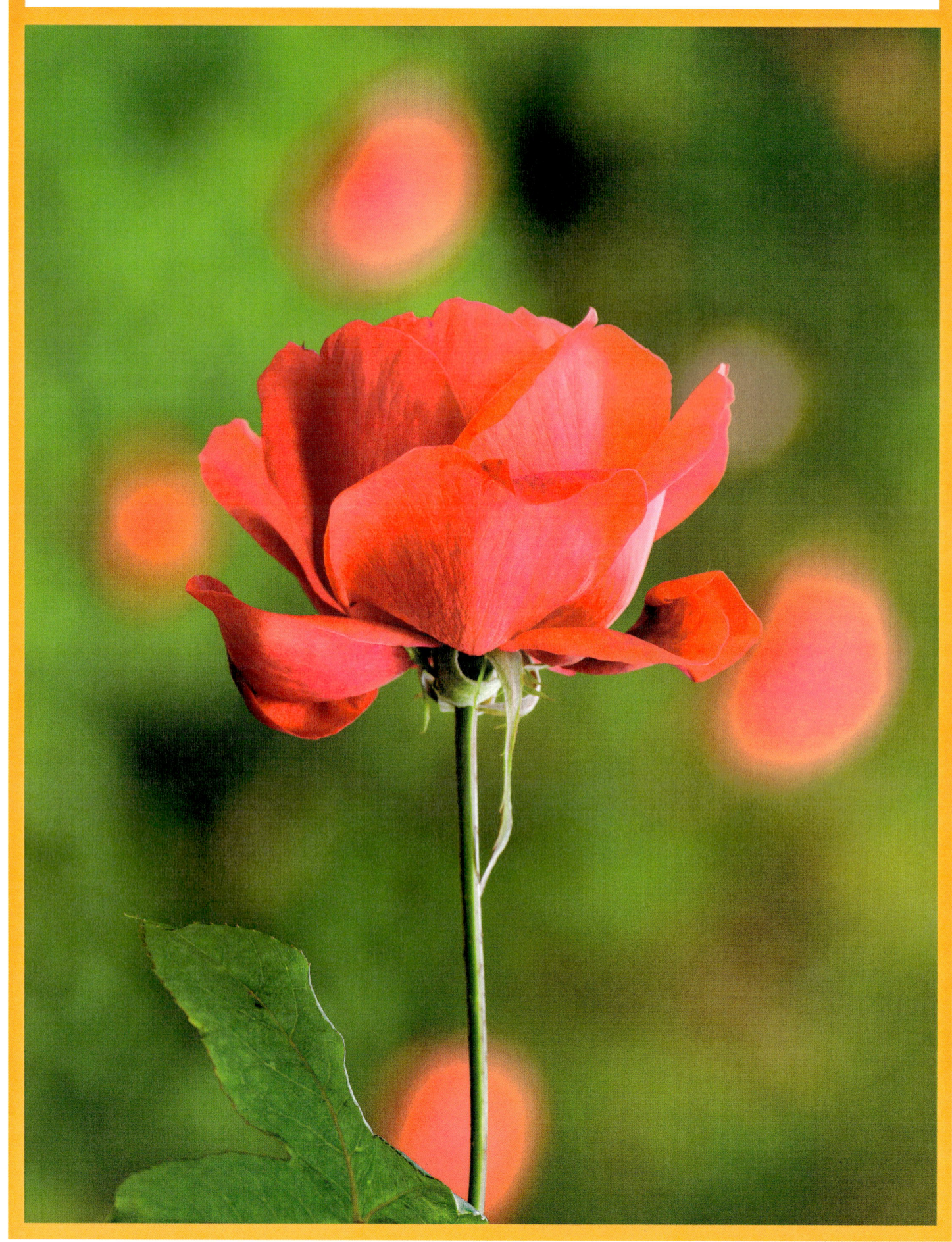

RED TORCH GINGER

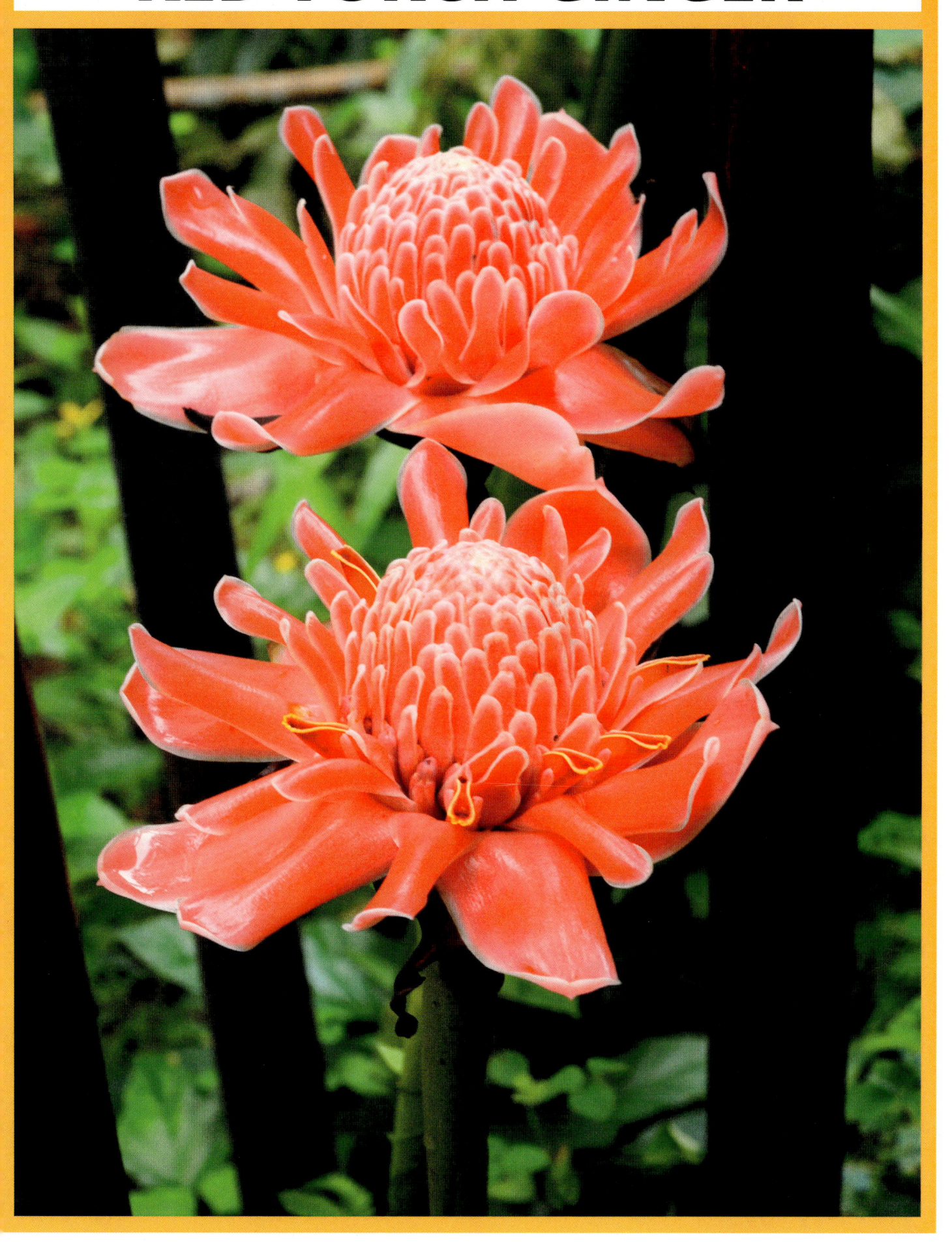

ROSE QUEEN IRIS

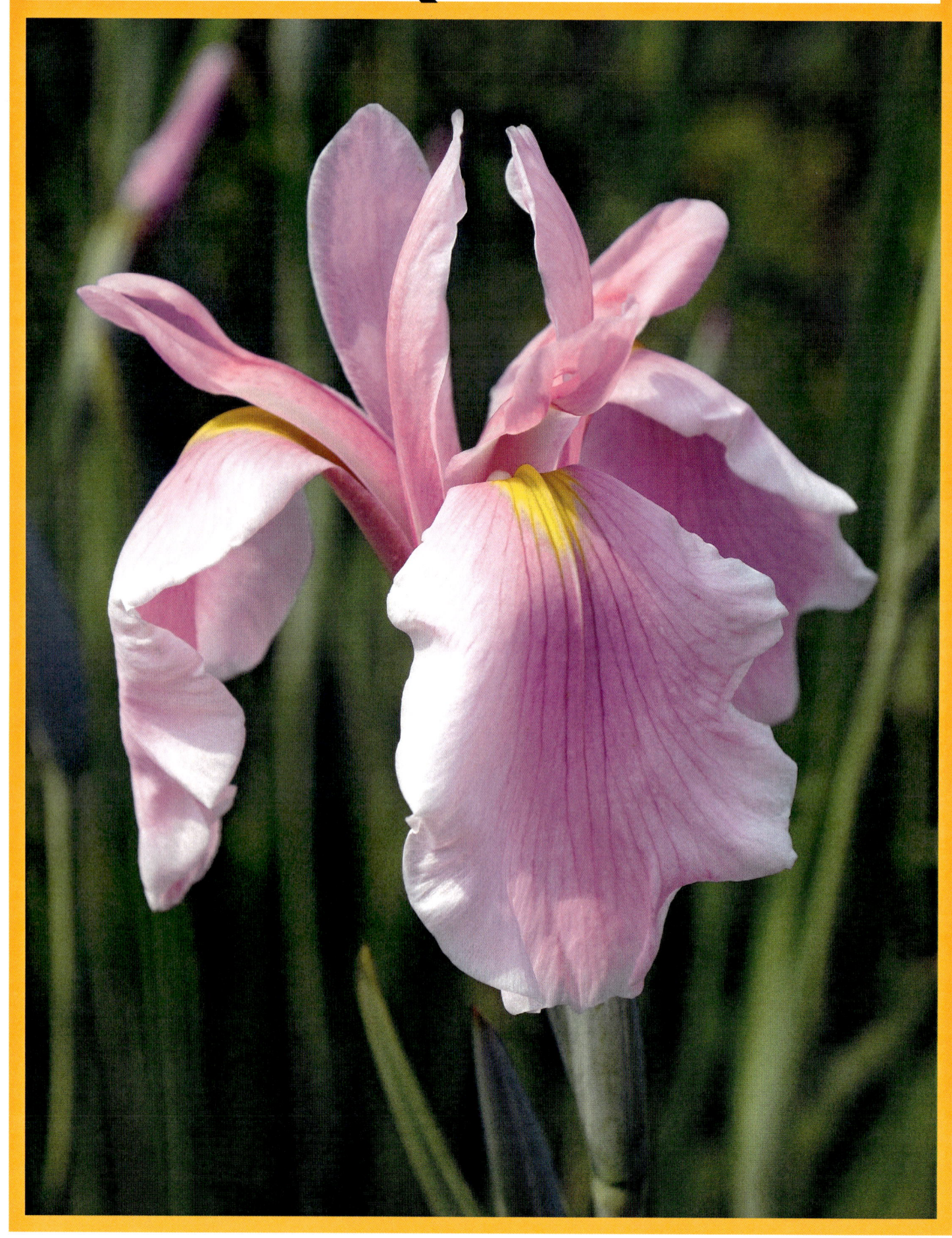

SNAPDRAGON

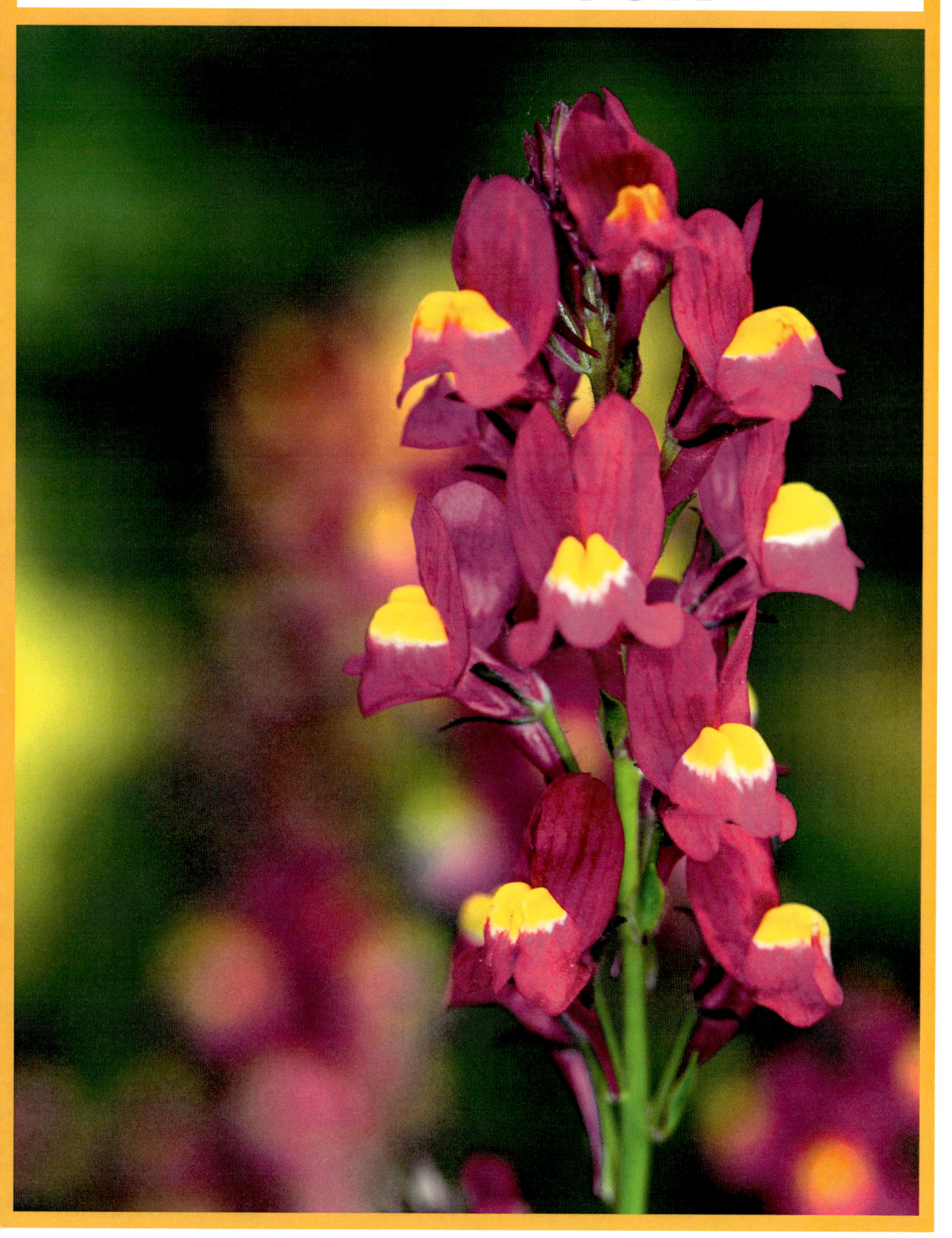

BIRD OF PARADISE

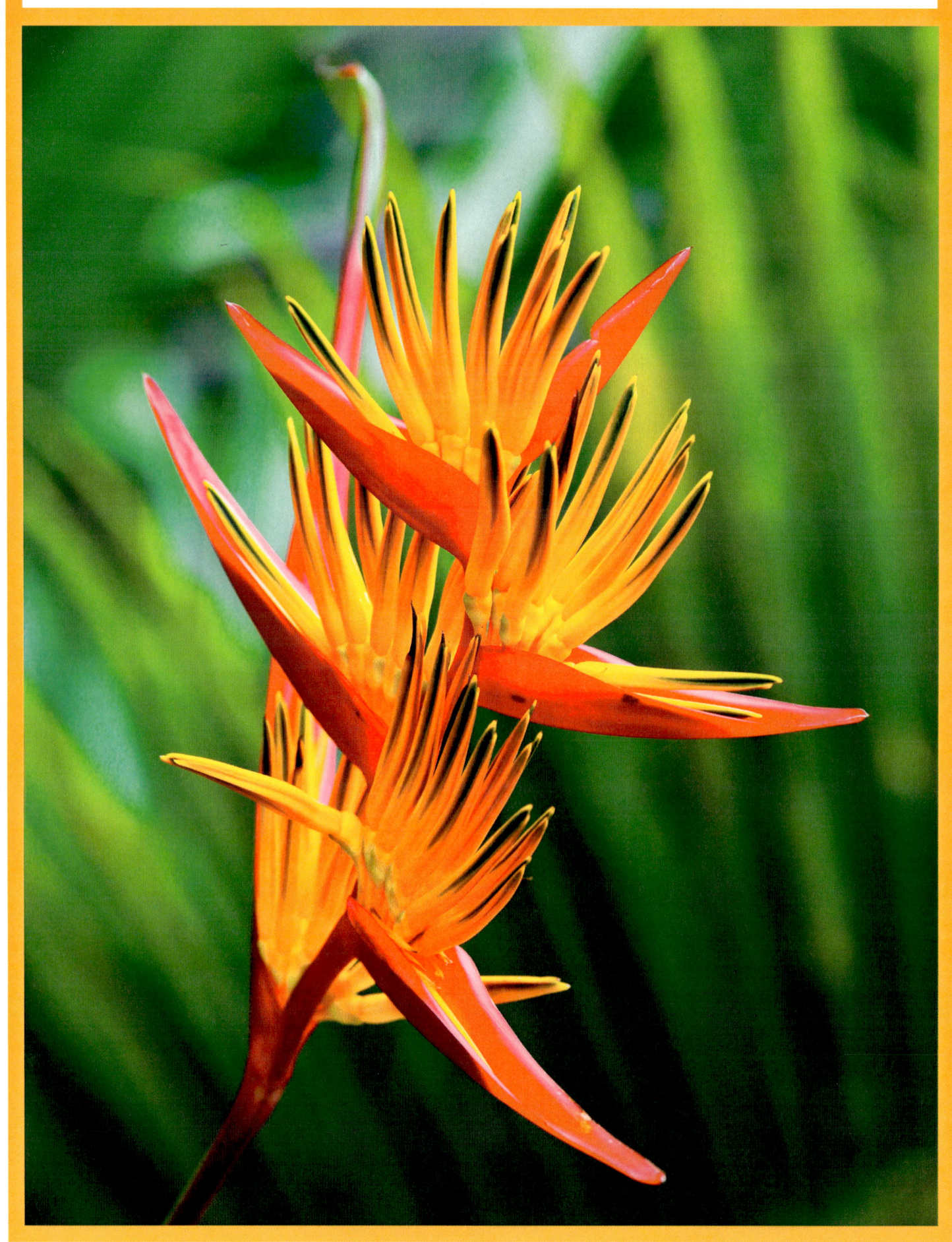

SUNFLOWER

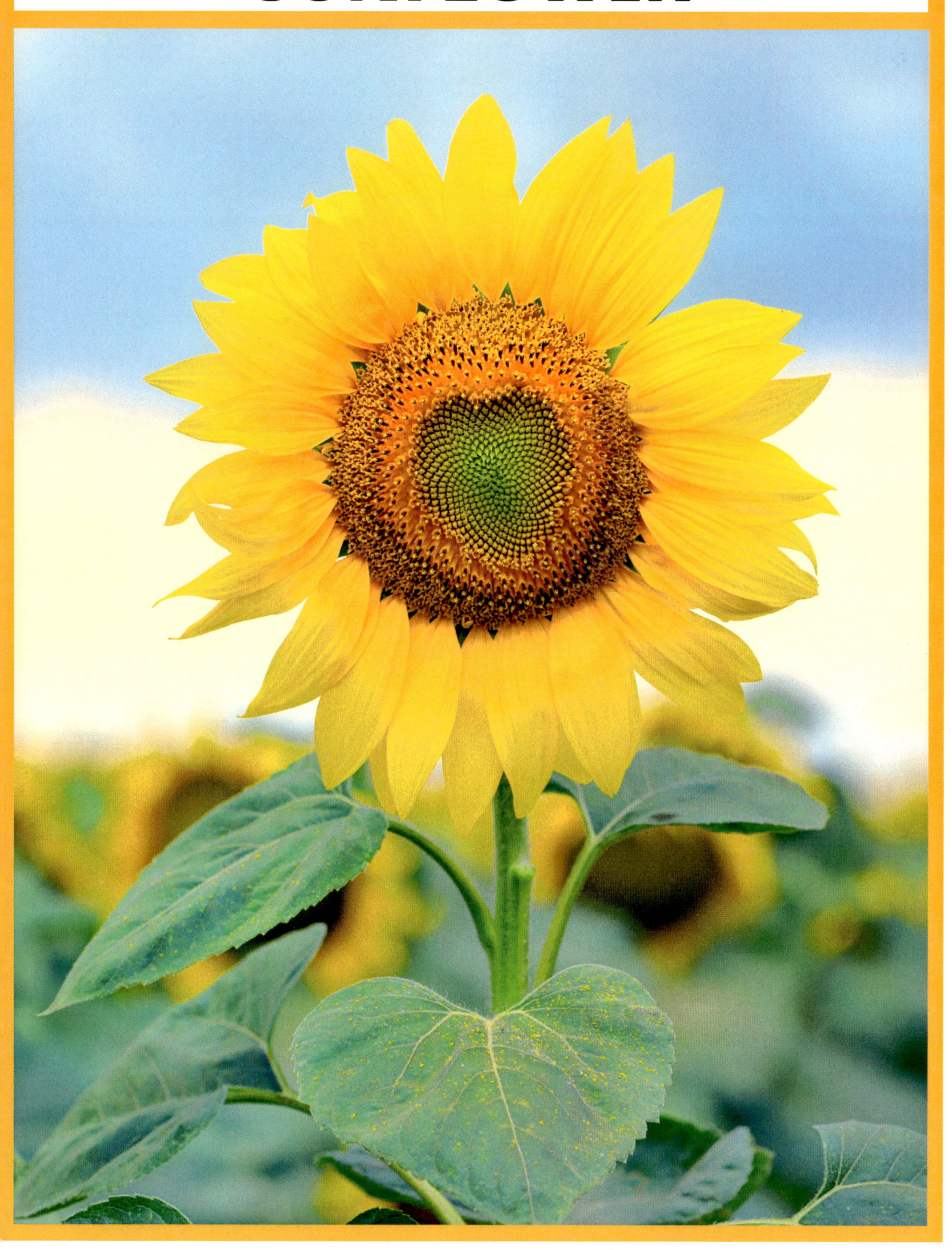

SWEET PEA FLOWER

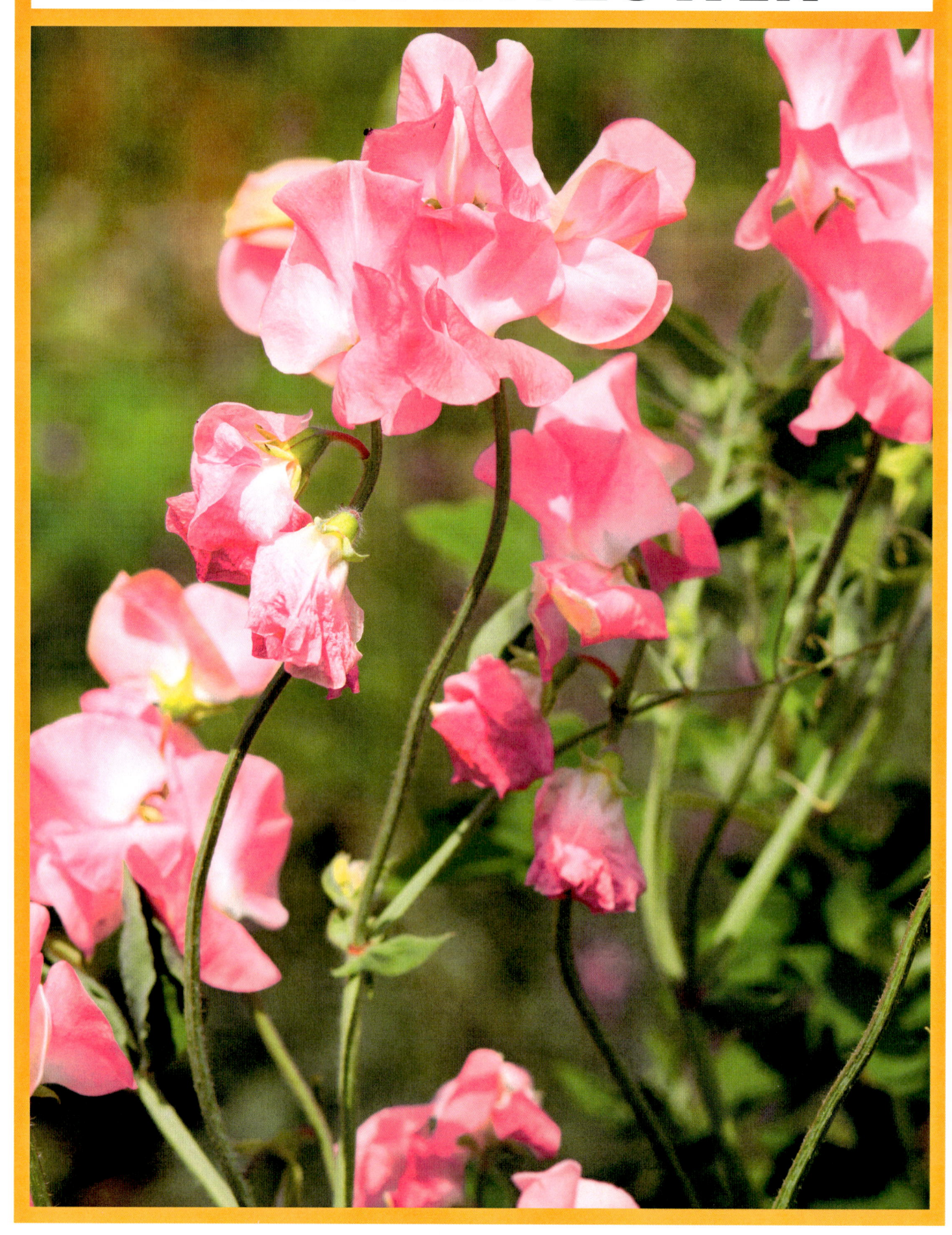

THISTLE FLOWER

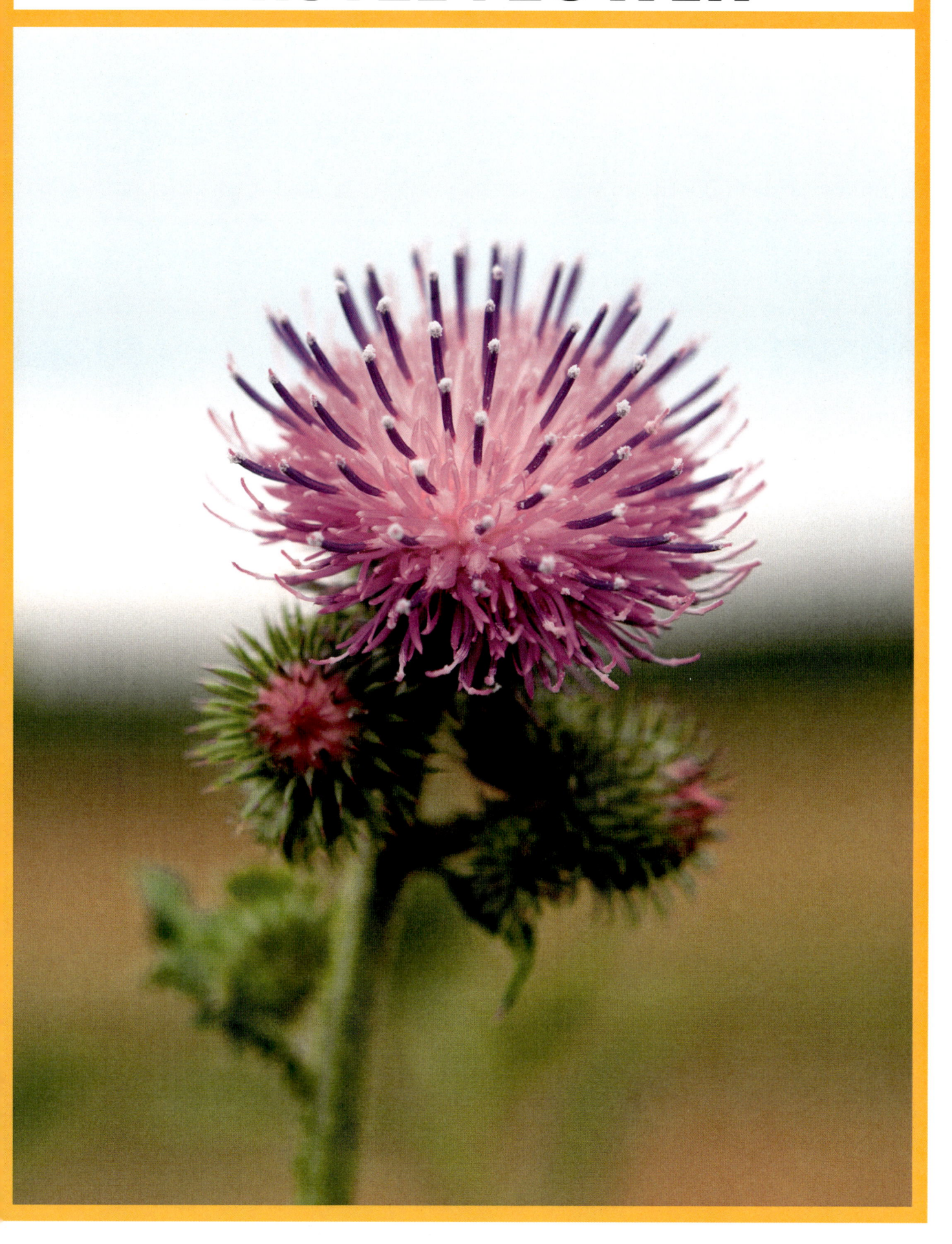

TULIP

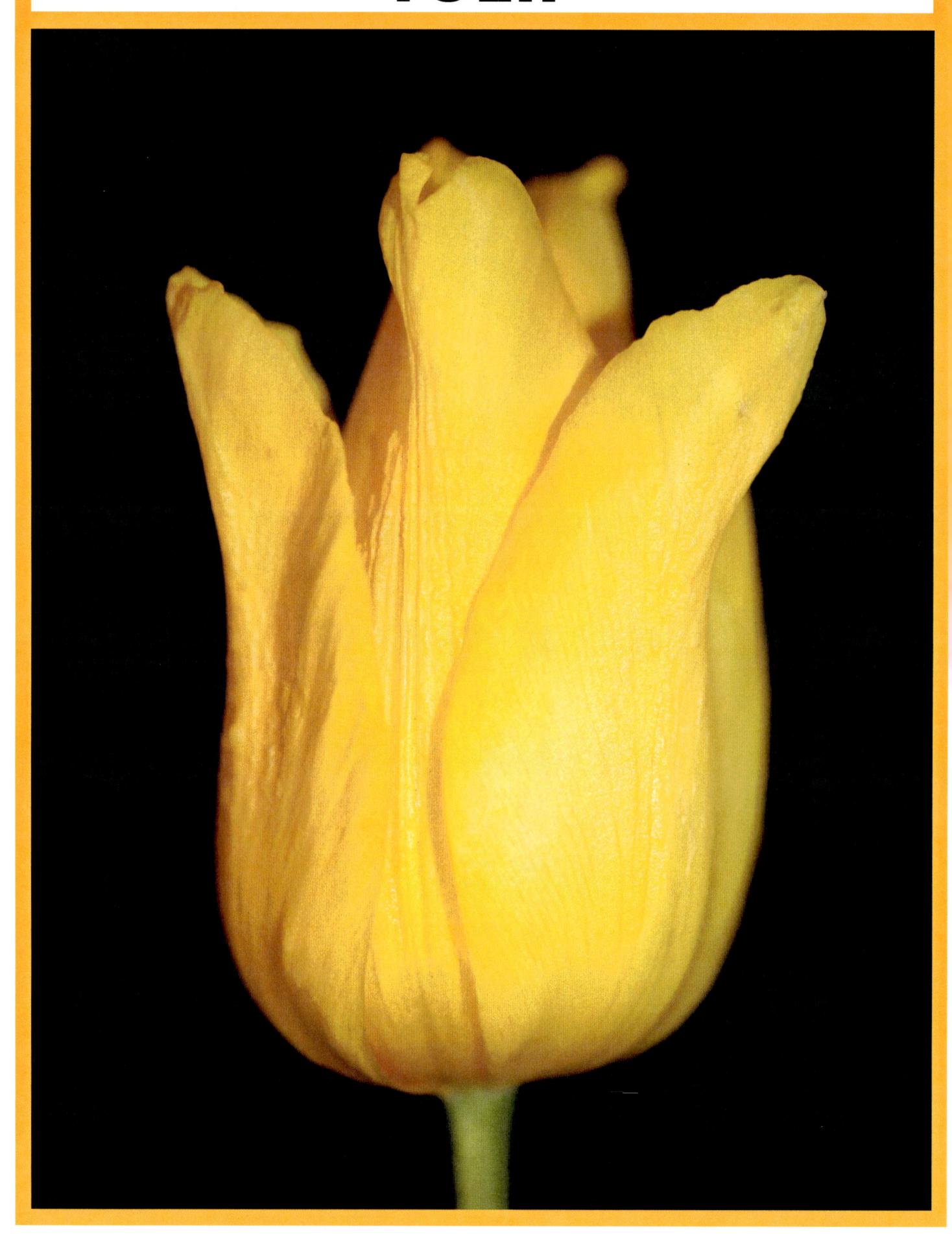

ORCHID

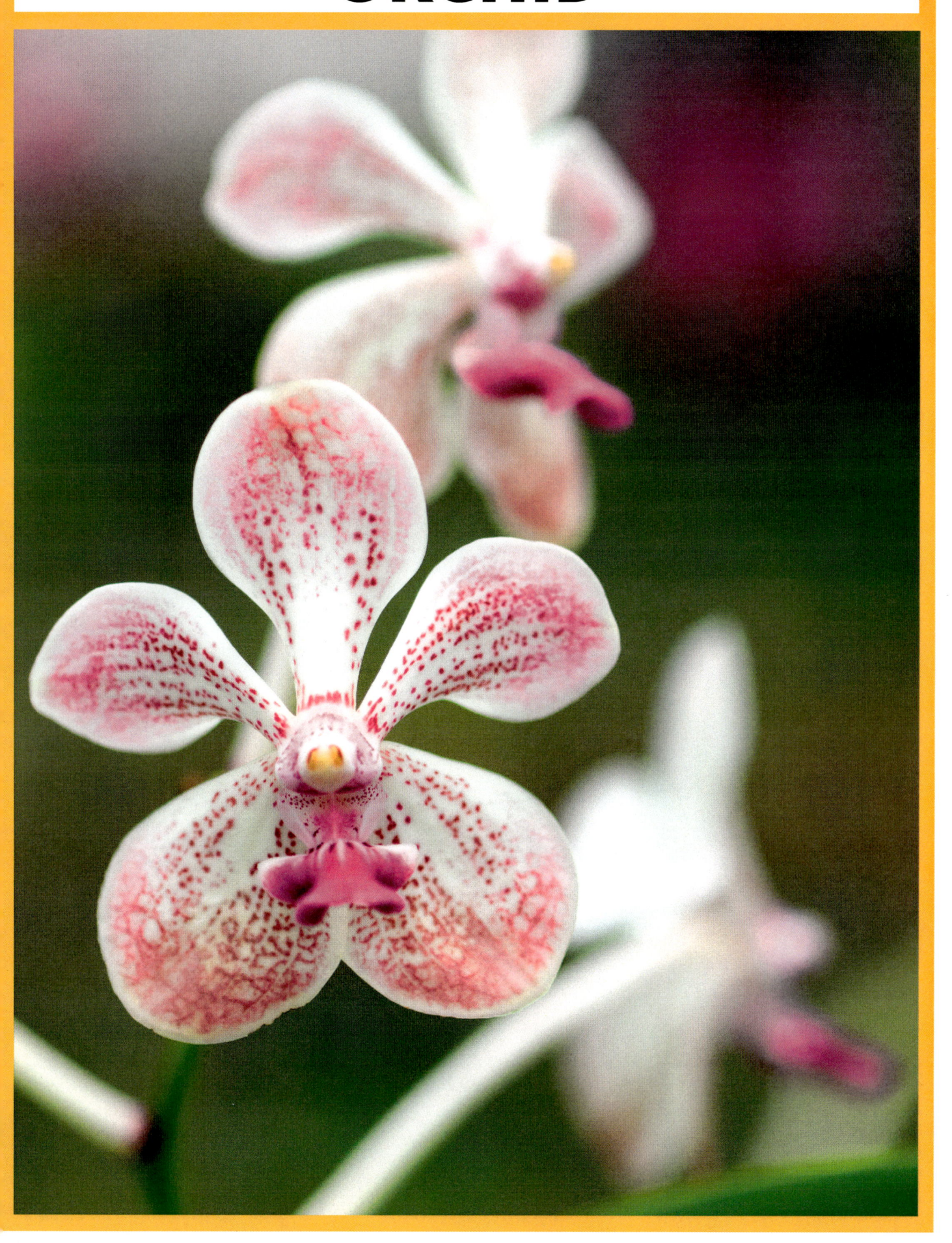

WHITE ANTHURIUM

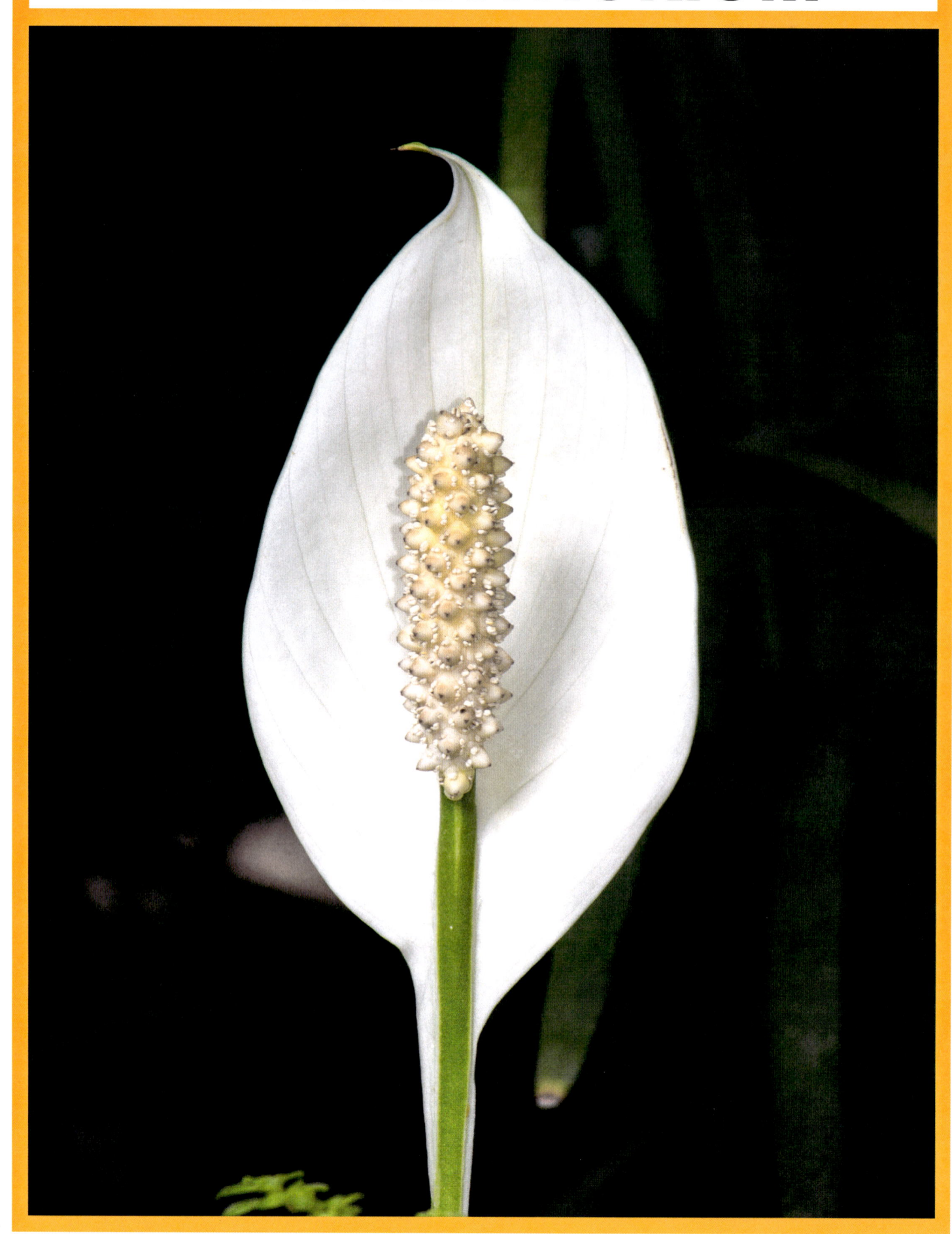

WHITE DAISY

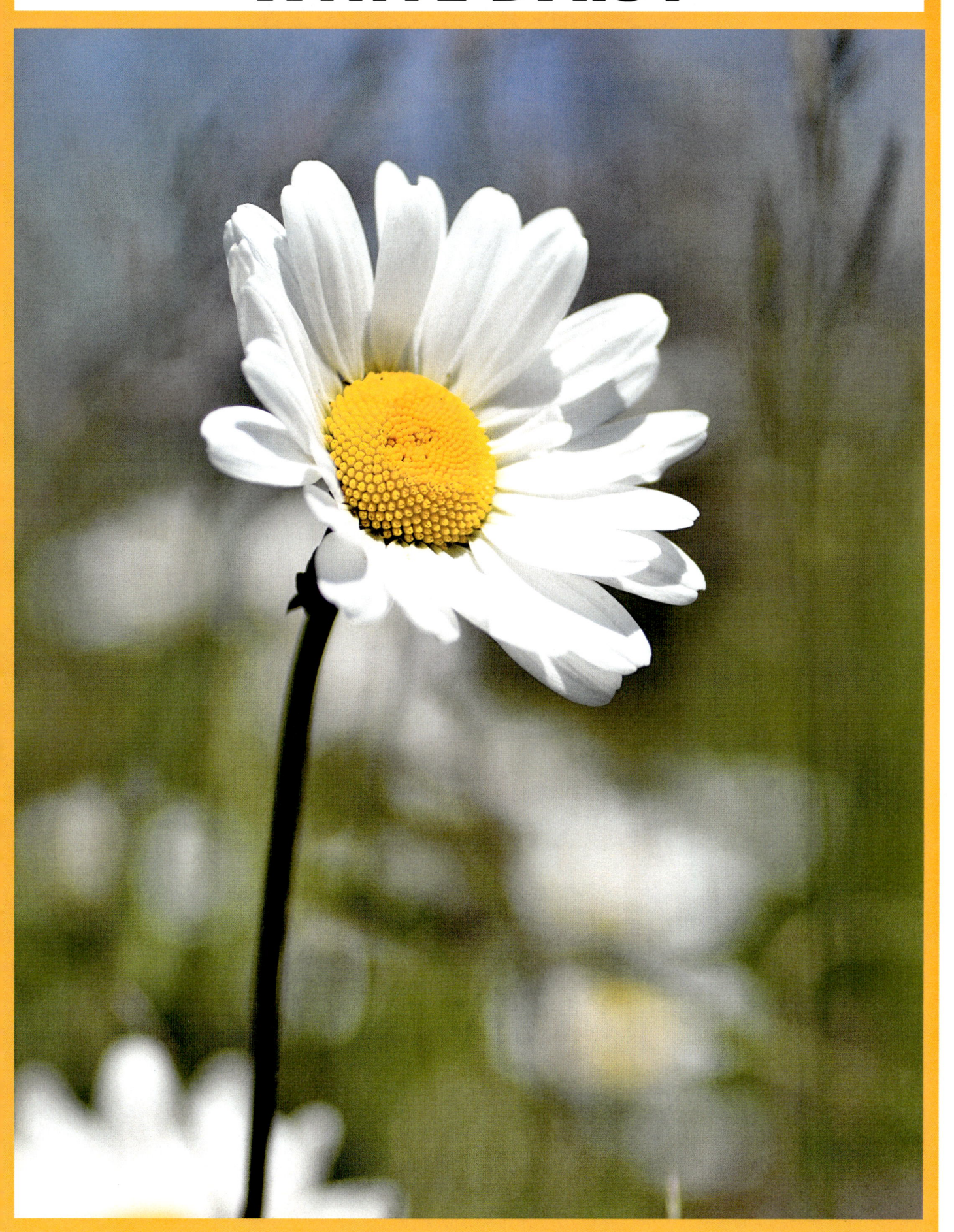

Made in United States
Orlando, FL
28 April 2022